MANUAL OF
ORTHOPAEDIC SURGERY

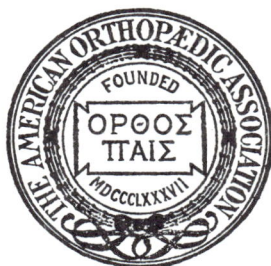

AMERICAN ORTHOPAEDIC ASSOCIATION

PREFACE TO THE FIFTH EDITION

In this fifth edition of the American Orthopaedic Association's Manual of Orthopaedic Surgery, several sections have been updated, notably the one on laboratory aids in orthopaedic management.

The manual is designed as a pocket source of basic information about this surgical specialty and the clinical and laboratory investigation of patients with orthopaedic complaints. Although it contains information of value to anyone dealing with such patients, it is aimed primarily toward medical students and residents beginning their orthopaedic experience and strives in a compact and readable form to provide a ready reference for use in the clinic or at the bedside.

The American Orthopaedic Association is deeply indebted to Dr. William F. Enneking and the members of his committee, Drs. Thomas D. Brower and Edgar L. Ralston, for updating this very useful little volume.

THORNTON BROWN, M.D.
President, American Orthopaedic Association

TABLE OF CONTENTS

THE HISTORY OF ORTHOPAEDIC SURGERY

Orthopaedic Surgery is a medical specialty that includes the investigation, preservation, restoration, and development of the form and function of the extremities, spine, and associated structures by medical, surgical and physical methods.

The term *"orthopaedia"* (orthos — straight, paidios — child) was first used by Nicholas Andrey in the title of a book, published in 1741, and devoted to a discussion of the deformities of the child. Subsequently this medical surgical specialty has grown to include problems of the adult and the acute derangements of the musculoskeletal system as well as the chronic.

Unlike the great infectious scourges that have swept the world in different ages, leaving no marks on any of the recovered remains of their victims to date their origins in antiquity, affections of the skeleton can be traced back to earliest man. The femur of *Java man,* Pithecanthropus erectus, dated approximately half a million years ago, demonstrates a mass of bone in its proximal portion that has been designated as an osteochondroma but probably represents reactive bone produced in response to local soft tissue and periosteal injury. Many of these ancient remains give ample evidence of man's pugnacity; skulls with depressed and fissured fractures and deep furrows from some type of axe or knife; and evidence of limbs having been hacked from the trunk. Later skeletons present injury from flint arrowheads with few portions of the body excepted. Some of these wounds show evidence of osseous healing while others with no evidence of reactive change suggest that death closely followed injury. The study of these skeletal remains also gives some suggestion of the crude splinting method that was used to support these fractured bones of the extremities. From the incidence of specific injuries seen in recovered skeletal parts, some idea of the industrial, social, and recreational activities of the ancient peoples can be obtained.

Although early man learned to care for fractured limbs by crude splinting, the first attempts at surgery were amputations as evidenced by bone stumps recovered from skeletons. Trephination of the skull must also rank with the most primitive of bone operations.

The first known written references to surgery of the skeleton are contained in such *Egyptian papyri* as the Ebers and the Edwin Smith, dated at about 1600 B.C. From Greece the *Hippocratic books,* dated between 400 B.C. and 100 A.D. *On Fractures, On Articulations,* and *On Surgery,* contain discussions of various types of fractures and the methods of treatment, including that of traction and immobilization by splinting and bandaging. The importance of early motion in the treatment of fractured extremities was emphasized. This was particularly true in reference to fractures and dislocations about the elbow joint where the tendency to contractures and ankylosis was apparently well recognized. The sections on the care of shoulder dislocations are of course classic and well-known. Congenital dislocation of the hip was recognized and the physical signs described. Detailed instructions for the treatment of club foot were listed. Spinal deformities were differentiated and well described. Open fractures were recognized as being potentially fatal and attempts were made to immediately reduce them and to splint them for longer periods than would be done for similar closed fractures.

Galen stands out as the great name in medicine and surgery in Rome. He may be designated the first of neuro-muscular physiologists, and made contributions to our knowledge of the circulatory system as well. He is the first individual known to have used the terms kyphosis, scoliosis, and lordosis, and to have advanced methods for the treatment of these deformities.

The Middle Ages are generally considered as the Dark Ages of medicine and surgery. Practitioners in general followed the precepts of Hippocrates and Galen, with a gradual deterioration of the original writings by repeated translations and addition of concepts, unsupported by adequate original observations, gradually covering and replacing the original writings. Some advances in the field of orthopaedic surgery were made, however, when *Paul of Aegina,* in the 7th century A.D., advised laminectomy for the relief of paralysis resulting from fracture of a vertebra. He also described a method for the treatment of fracture of the patella and advised the cutting of bone with a chisel in the correction of malunion following fracture. In the universities at Salerno and Bologna the study of anatomy was revived during the 12th and 13th centuries although animals apparently were used in dissection. *Guy de Chauliac* at the University of Montpelier in the 14th century, advised continuous traction over a pulley for fractures of the femur.

With the flowering of the Renaissance the study of human anatomy was reintroduced. The work of *Leonardo da Vinci* in his drawings of human dissections gave impetus for further study as well as offering the direct value of these original observations. The age of the great anatomists followed. About this time medical and surgical services for field armies was introduced with the confidence that the application of the newer knowledge of anatomy would provide for better care of the injured. Among the more famous of the military surgeons was *Pare,* whose greatest contribution was the advocacy of the suture over the cautery in amputations. He also advised laminectomy for the relief of cord compression following fractures of the vertebrae. Military surgeons, who attended the field hospitals of the day, had at their disposal the armourers who, under guidance of the surgeons, designed the first functional prostheses.

The 17th century brought the modern era of medicine and surgery with such names as Leewenhoek, Harvey, and Sydenham leading the way in the investigation of special areas. Spinal curvature, gibbus, gout and other arthritides, rickets, scurvy, and congenital deformities were described and treatment advocated. *Havers* of London gave the first histological description of bone with the result that his name is linked with the vascular canals in bone.

During the 18th century orthopaedic surgery was established as a branch of medicine and surgery, with the construction of hospitals for the treatment of skeletal deformity and disease. The design of braces and supports for the treatment of these varied disorders reached a new height in ingenuity. The studies of *Belchier, Duhamel,* and *John Hunter* laid the foundation for the studies on bone growth that have continued down to the present time.

In addition to the introduction of detailed scientific study of the skeletal and muscular systems, this century also saw the introduction of new surgical methods. Joint resection for infection was introduced and in some cases supplanted amputation. Tendon surgery was also introduced for the first time. During this century the name of *Percival Potts* became known for his discussion of fractures and paralysis from spinal disease. This was also the century of John Hunter whose influence on surgery extends to the present time. He was interested in the study of the reparative process of all body tissues. He was able to record personal observations following the rupture of his own Achilles tendon, suffered at the age of 40 while dancing. As a result of his experiments in bone growth, Hunter became the first to recognize the dynamic character of the skeletal system, with growth occurring in one portion and absorption following in another.

These pioneers of the 18th century and those preceding them laid the groundwork for extensive studies of the skeletal system in the 19th and 20th centuries. Analysis of bone growth, bone repair, and calcification proceeded together with studies of the gross and miscroscopic anatomy of bone and joint affection. With the advent of anesthesia and the introduction of asepsis, rapid advances were made in the open surgical correction of orthopaedic affections.

The surgical principles of John Hunter were brought to America shortly after the Revolution by *Philip Syng Physick.* After studying with Hunter for 4 years, he returned to Philadelphia in 1792 and in 1805 became the first Professor of Surgery at the University of Pennsylvania. A pupil of Physick, *John Rhea Barton,* performed the first known arthroplasty on an ankylosed hip joint in 1826.

William Detmold, a pupil of the German surgeon, Stromeyer, came to New York City in 1837 and four years later was appointed surgeon of the Bellevue Hospital. He was thus able to introduce German orthopaedic surgical methods to this country. Another German surgeon, *Louis Bauer,* settled in New York in 1852. Teaching at the Medical and Surgical Institution, he published in 1864 his lectures on orthopaedic surgery. *Valentine Mott,* Professor of Surgery at the College of Physicians and Surgeons, was interested in orthopaedic surgery and in 1843 published *Orthopaedia,* describing both operative and mechanical surgery. He persuaded *James Knight* to specialize in orthopaedic surgery and in 1863, under Dr. Knight's direction, the New York Society for the Relief of the Ruptured and Crippled was founded with the hospital established in Dr. Knight's home. This institution continues today as the Hospital for Special Surgery. *Lewis Sayre,* another of the pioneer orthopaedic surgeons of New York, advocated the use of the plaster of Paris jacket for the treatment of scoliosis and tuberculosis of the spine. He had organized the orthopaedic clinic at Bellevue Hospital and became the first American to receive the title of Professor of Orthopaedic Surgery. *Charles Fayette Taylor,* another pioneer in New York, is recognized for the spinal brace he devised for the treatment of tuberculosis and for the establishment, with Theodore Roosevelt, Sr., of the New York Orthopaedic Dispensary and Hospital. *Henry G. Davis* of New York was among the first to devise and use continuous traction for the correction of deformity of bones and joints.

In Boston, *Dr. John Ball Brown,* Consultant Surgeon to the Massachusetts General Hospital, founded in 1833 a private hospital, The Boston Orthopaedic Institution or Hospital for the Cure of Deformities of the Human Frame. A contemporary, *Henry Bigelow,* is credited with performing the first hip excision in America and described a technique for correction of hip flexion contracture by subcutaneous tenotomy. *Buckminster Brown,* a son of John Ball Brown, was one of the first to devote his practice exclusively to orthopaedics and organized a private hospital, the House of the Good Samaritan. He established and endowed a Chair of Orthopaedic Surgery at Harvard Medical School. Succeeding Brown as visiting orthopaedist at the Good Samaritan was *Edward Bradford.* Bradford was later joined there and at the Children's Hospital by *Robert Lovett.* British and American orthopaedic surgery were once again combined when Lovett joined *Sir Robert Jones* in producing a new text on orthopaedic surgery. Robert Jones, the father of modern orthopaedic surgery, had worked for 11 years with his uncle, *Hugh Owen Thomas,* in Liverpool and he continued to teach and refine the principles that this pioneer orthopaedic surgeon had followed in his busy practice. In the first World War, Robert Jones was selected to head the orthopaedic service of the British Army. His organization of that service and the results accomplished in the treatment of the injured in the Army brought him and his specialty world-wide recognition. Joining with Lovett in the publication of *Orthopaedic Surgery,* the best in practice on both sides of the Atlantic became available to all interested in this specialty. Following the Second World War this collaboration was broadened to include the publication of the *Journal of Bone and Joint Surgery* jointly by the American and British Orthopaedic Associations.

The American Orthopaedic Association was founded in 1887 with Virgil P. Gibney the first president. Two years later the Association published its first Transactions, continued to the present as the Journal of Bone and Joint Surgery. World War I provided American surgeons extensive experience in the treatment of wounds of soft tissues, bones, and joints and gave great impetus to the development of orthopaedic surgery as a specialty. Although Lewis Sayre, at Bellevue Medical College, had been the first American to receive the title of Professor of Orthopaedic Surgery in 1861, World War I and the years following saw the organization of orthopaedic services and in most medical schools the formation of orthopaedic departments or sections, offering opportunities for postgraduate study. In increasing numbers the graduates of these programs joined the general medical community. In 1932 the *American Academy of Orthopaedic Surgeons* was organized and the first of its annual meetings was held in 1933. This organization has now grown to be the largest orthopaedic organization in the world, influencing all aspects of the practice and teaching of the specialty. Recognizing the need for the establishment of certain standards in the practice of the specialty, the *American Board of Orthopaedic Surgery* was organized in 1934, and examinations have been held yearly for candidates who wish to present themselves for certification by the Board. World War II and the years afterward saw a further increase in programs and positions for graduate training. To maintain satisfactory standards of education these programs are under scrutiny of the Residency Review Committee of the American Medical Association, the American Board of Orthopaedic Surgery, and the American Academy of Orthopaedic Surgeons.

During World War II the Surgeon General of the Army appointed *Sterling Bunnell* consultant to the Army for hand surgery. Special hospital centers for hand surgery were established throughout the country for the care of military patients with these special problems. Following the war, this group of surgeons formed the *American Society for Surgery of the Hand,* made Sterling Bunnell its president and in 1947 held the first of its annual meetings.

In 1948 a group of young orthopaedic surgeons from Great Britain toured centers in the United States. The next year a group from the United States and Canada sponsored by the American and the Canadian Orthopaedic Associations toured Great Britain. This *Exchange Fellowship* has now become an established program and has given leadership in educational programs in all of the countries involved. In 1949 the *Association of Bone and Joint Surgeons* was organized. In 1953 it initiated and has since supported the publication, *Clinical Orthopaedics and Related Research.* In 1954 the *Orthopaedic Research Society* was organized and has held its meeting annually in conjunction with the meeting of the Academy. At about this same time under the leadership of A.R. Shands, Jr., the *Orthopaedic Research and Education Foundation* was established. This organization has played an important role in initiating and supporting, through financial grants, the research and educational projects which have benefited the specialty.

The past decades have seen the strengthening and the maturation of organizations and educational structures in orthopaedic surgery throughout the United States. Satisfactory as these advances may be, the scientific progress has been even more remarkable. The introduction of penicillin markedly changed the picture of osteomyelitis just as streptomycin and other anti-tuberculous drugs changed that of tuberculosis of the bones and joints, and poliomyelitis vaccine eliminated the problem of this disease. However, problems of acute injury in our age of speed and of degenerative disease of the skeletal system in our expanding elder population continue to mount and demand solution. A better understanding of the metabolic processes of bone, cartilage and soft tissue through research and the refinement of technical procedures in surgical and physiological rehabilitation promise solution of some of these problems. Experience from the past, however, would suggest that as these solutions are found, other problems will appear and present new challenges to the orthopaedic surgeon of the future.

ORTHOPAEDIC HISTORY TAKING

An accurate history is frequently of critical importance in early diagnosis and later may be an important factor when a decision as to therapy is being made. Although the patient's chief complaint may seem to indicate a condition that refers exclusively to the musculoskeletal system, it is a mistake to indicate that there is such a thing as an orthopaedic history. The history in seemingly even the most straightforward case of isolated skeletal injury should be complete in all medical relationships. Neither the history nor the physical examination should focus on a broken limb to the exclusion of the other body systems. The history should include the entire person although it is apparent that in emergency situations the less obvious historical features may be obtained and recorded after proper emergency procedures have been instituted.

The chief complaint should indicate the symptom or symptoms from which the patient seeks relief. It may often be best to state this in the patient's own words.

PRESENT ILLNESS

Certain features of the history should be emphasized in the patient whose complaints involve primarily the musculoskeletal system.

A. Injury: Whether recent or old the history of an injury should include the how, what, when and where. 1) the *how* will list all of the features that may be of interest to the surgeon at the time of treatment or later and does not concern itself only with what may be of interest legally. 2) The *what* records the patient's description of the injury. 3) The *when* indicates an exact calendar date, if not an exact hour, and is never adequately answered by "two weeks ago" or "last winter." This fact becomes increasingly important in today's involvement in the judicial assessment of medical or injury liability. 4) The *where* should state

9

just that and in the words that will convey the intended description clearly even when reread some years later.

B. Onset: A clear understanding of the onset of the symptom or symptoms is demanded.

1. Was the onset immediate with an overpowering systemic reaction or was it insidious and gradual in appearance? Was it associated with any known specific activity or was it completely unrelated to any activity?

2. What were the associated systemic symptoms, if any? Has there been temperature elevation or chills and sweats? Has there been associated general fatigue, malaise or weight loss?

C. Pain: Pain must be described with specific characteristics.

1. *Location.* The exact location, as the patient indicates, is always noted. Is hip pain located in the proximal thigh or over the ilium or sacroiliac joint?

2. *Character.* Dull, aching, sharp or intense?

3. *Severity.* Has it been severe enough to interrupt work and daily activities?

4. *Relief.* Does it improve with rest? Does heat alleviate it? Has any medication been noted to give some relief?

5. *Aggravation.* Is it worse with activity? If so, what specific activity? Coughing? Sneezing? Is it worse when standing than when walking?

6. *Daily variation.* Is it worse on arising in the morning and then eased during the usual daily activities? Is it worse or better at night? Has it ever awakened the person from sleep?

7. *Radiation.* Is the pain always sharply localized or does it at times radiate from a focus to other parts of the body? Do certain types of activity initiate this? Is there any other pain elsewhere in the body seemingly related or unrelated?

8. *Course.* Is it getting worse or better? Has any treatment been tried and what effect may it have had?

D. Deformity:

1. *Time.* When was the deformity first noted? Recently or is it long-standing? Was it associated with injury or dissease?

2. *Change.* Has it improved or has it advanced over a certain period of time?

3. *Character.* Is it associated with swelling or inflammation locally? Is it associated with joint stiffness?

4. *Disability.* How much does it interfere with normal activities?

5. *Inheritance.* Is there a familial incidence?

6. *Past treatment.*

E. Paralysis:

1. *Time of onset.* Was the paralysis immediate or gradual in development? Was it associated with any systemic symptoms, disease or injury?

2. *Extent.* Portions of trunk and/or extremities involved?

3. *Progress or regression.*

4. *Associated sensory disturbances.* Paresthesias, hypo- or hyperesthesias? Is it associated with pain, headache, or backache?

5. *Sphincter control.*

6. *Disability.* Has it interfered with normal activities?

7. *Past treatment.*

REVIEW OF SYSTEMS

A complete systemic review should be included. A great number of patients treated on a general orthopaedic service are aged and are likely to have abnormalities other than and unassociated with the musculoskeletal complaint. All positive responses should be developed as to time of onset of symptoms, duration, past treatment, and present status including any present medication with exact dosages recorded. As many of these patients may later undergo a surgical procedure requiring general anesthesia, inquiry as to the status of the cardiorespiratory system, the urinary system, the neurological system, and the gastrointestinal system, should be complete.

PAST MEDICAL HISTORY

This should include:

1. *General condition of health* with notation of any weight loss or gain.

2. *Past diseases, injuries, and operations* including dates, treatment, complications and present status.

3. *Habits.* Alcohol, tobacco and drugs.

4. A statement should be recorded as to the *presence or absence of drug sensitivity and present medications.*

5. *Military history.*

FAMILY HISTORY

A thorough review of the family history is important not only because of the genetic relationships of certain musculo-skeletal defects, but also because of other associated or nonassociated defects. These relationships are probably more important to the epidemiologist or the geneticist today than are the more traditionally sought family relationships that in the past might have given some clue to the origin of a musculoskeletal disease such as tuberculosis. Much remains to be learned of the genetic relationships of club foot, scoliosis, and other developmental abnormalities and this will be possible only by the development of a complete and thorough review of each disease process as it affects *families.*

SOCIAL, ECONOMIC, INDUSTRIAL HISTORY

This portion of the history is one of the most important aspects of the history of the patient with a musculoskeletal complaint. Patients with musculoskeletal disease and deformity notably remain under treatment for long periods of time so that the social and economic factors become prominent features that may go completely unnoticed in a more acute disease process. If the patient is in the younger age group, family relationships and educational requirements must be well understood to allow for these and perhaps associated emotional adjustments that may have to be made during the long periods of treatment and convalescence. If the patient is in the middle or wage-earning years of life, the economic impact of prolonged treatment must be understood by the physician. If the patient's work requires any amount of physical activity, his physician must gain intimate knowledge of these requirements so that the return to work may be planned and adjusted as the needs require. These features of the history should be recorded early in the treatment process so that insurance liability, workmen's compensation, and other economic features are as familiar to the physician as are the changes noted on repeated reviewing of x-ray films of some specific injury.

If the patient is elderly, family relationships and the available facilities for long-term and perhaps terminal care must be considered. Such information as does the patient live in a house or apartment, who will be with him, are there stairs to climb, and other aspects of the home environment should be considered early in the treatment process and not delayed to the day before the planned discharge from the hospital. All of these features of the patient's complex historical background require complete physician involvement if recovery is to be expected under optimum conditions and in the shortest time.

ORTHOPAEDIC PHYSICAL EXAMINATION

A. GENERAL EXAMINATION

Certain portions of the physical examination of the musculoskeletal system will be discussed on a regional basis—that is, the ankle, the hip, etc., as specific methods are used in these particular regions. Other portions of the physical examination are applicable to all the regions of the musculoskeletal system and will be described in this introductory section. The topics to be covered in this general section are the gait, muscle power, measurements of joint motion, determination of limb length, and examination of injured extremities. As each of these topics is discussed, its relevance will be pointed out by the common clinical examples.

1. Gait, Posture and Deformities

Many conditions of the musculoskeletal system will be brought to the physician's attention because of abnormalities in gait. In order to appreciate these abnormalities, it is well to become familiar with normal gait. It is useful when the patient presents himself for examination to observe him walking and/or standing, as well as arising from a chair prior to disrobing for examination. During these periods of time, patients are generally unaware that they are being observed and will present their activities in their usual fashion. Frequently patients, and particularly children, when disrobed in front of an audience will walk in an unnatural fashion and deprive the examining physician of a useful observation. The specific things one looks for during this observation are the presence of deformities, objective evidence of discomfort, evidence of muscle weakness or joint stiffness, lack of coordination, and specific patterns of gait associated with various disease states. After these unguarded observations have been made, the patient is disrobed and his stance, posture, and gait are scrutinized in some detail. The common deformities one may see with the patient standing are an increased roundness of the normal thoracic curve of the spine called a *kyphosis*.

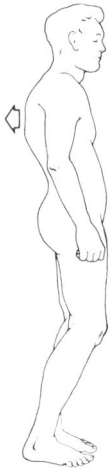

Fig. 1
Kyphosis

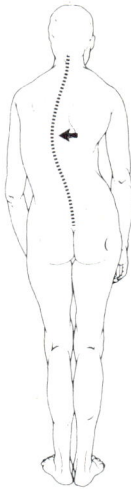

Fig. 2
Scoliosis

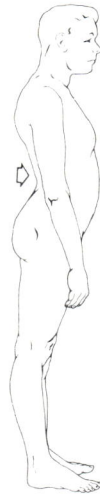

Fig. 3
Lordosis

a marked lateral deformity of the spine termed a *scoliosis*, or a marked increase in the normal lumbar curve referred to as *lordosis*.

Obvious differences in length and circumference of the extremities are noted at this time as are other gross deformities such as bowing of the legs, termed *genu varus,* or knock-knees, termed *genu valgus.*

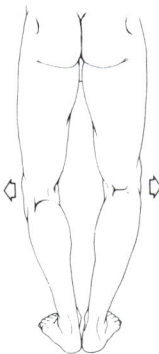

Fig. 4 Genu varus

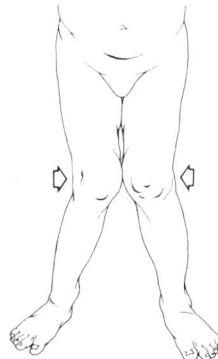

Fig. 5 Genu valgus

The terms *varus* and *valgus* are frequently used in the description of musculoskeletal deformities. They refer specifically to the direction in which the apex of the deformity lies in relationship to the midline. If the apex of the deformity points away from the midline, it is termed a varus deformity, whereas if the apex of the deformity is directly toward the midline, it is termed a valgus deformity. You will note in the illustration showing a genu varus that the apex of the deformity is at the knee, hence the term genu, and that the apex of the deformity points away from the midline of the extremity. The reverse is true in the illustration of genu valgus. Thus the terms varus and valgus are used in any region of the body to describe the direction of the deformity. Other terms used to describe various regions are *coxa*—the hip, *pes*—the foot, and *cubitus*—the elbow. Although these deformities will be examined in detail later on in the physical examination, they are generally first appreciated and noted during this general part of the examination. More specific descriptions and methods of examination of these deformities will be found under the regional portion of the examination.

When the patient's posture is examined, it is well to ask him to walk as naturally as he can and observe his gait both from the side and either in front or behind. Generally one can get a fairly objective estimate of pain during this part of the examination and associate it with the description of the patient's subjective complaints of pain obtained during the history. This correlation of the two findings frequently gives the physician insight into some of the motives and/or disability of the patient. When the patient limps because of pain, it is called an *"antalgic gait."* This is best typified by the timing of the gait, that is, when the patient steps on the painful extremity, he will remove his weight as quickly as possible and will walk as if he had a thorn in his foot or a stone in his shoe. This quick component of weight-bearing on a painful extremity is more reliable than facial grimacing or other indications of pain. Not infrequently patients who are *malingering* will exaggerate limps when they are aware they are being observed, thus it is necessary to observe their gait when they are unaware of the observation.

Usually weakness, when present, will be one of the patient's presenting complaints and it may first be observed during the general part of the examination. It is more thoroughly evaluated during the determination of muscle power (see below) and during the detailed examination of the various anatomic regions. However, when patients present with limps as their complaint observation of locomotion carefully noting the timing of the gait, may frequently distinguish between a limp of pain and a limp of weakness. In contrast to antalgic limp gaits, limps of weakness are manifested by the "quick" component of the gait on the unaffected extremity. With muscle weakness the patient usually must balance on the weakened extremity and, in order to do this, will spend more time on this extremity than on an unaffected extremity.

Similarly, joint stiffness is usually called to the physician's attention during the history, but again the degree to which the stiffness may be disabling is more apparent during this general part of the examination. While stiffness or loss of joint motion, as with weakness, is usually first noted during this part of the examination, it is evaluated in more detail as specific joints are examined during the regional part of the examination. It is well to be aware that patients who are being evaluated for compensable disability may exaggerate their stiffness, particularly when they are aware that it is being evaluated. Many times it is helpful to note the general ranges of motion during this part of the examination and compare them with those obtained during the regional portions of the examination when the patient's attention is called to specific joints.

Incoordinate motions may very well be first noted during this portion of the examination. The lack of coordination, which may seriously interfere with the patient's function, may be due to combinations of weakness, stiffness, and/or the inability to coordinate the joint and muscle function. As these are being noted by the examiner during the general part of the examination, it may be well to ask the patient to perform specific functions of daily living, such as dressing, opening and closing doors, moving furniture, etc., to gain some general impression of the level of disability prior to regional examination.

Also at this time in the examination, specific gait abnormalities that fall into a rather characteristic pattern of a particular lesion may be noted. Frequently these patterns will direct attention to specific anatomic regions for more detailed evaluation. Thus, the patient whose presenting complaint is "I don't walk right," may, by the pattern of gait he exhibits, direct the examiner's attention to his hip when he demonstrates a "gluteus medius" swaying-type of limp denoting hip instability. It is well to caution the inexperienced examiner who, following the completion of history taking, has his nurse place the disrobed patient on the examining table that he may be misled by the vagaries of patient's complaints and spend most of his time examining the wrong region. He is thus left with a rather puzzling assembly of historical and physical findings, when in fact observation of the patient's gait and posture would indicate accurately where attention is to be focused.

2. Crutches, Canes and Braces

Many patients when seen for the first time will be using various devices to assist them in walking. These would include canes, crutches, braces or walkers. These assists are used generally for one of two purposes; that is, either to relieve discomfort by lessening the weight-bearing on a painful extremity or to provide additional stability to permit function. A third, less frequent use is to assist in maintaining balance.

Relief from Weight-bearing: It is well to understand some of the mechanics of normal weight-bearing joints, before considering the part that canes and crutches play in the relief of weight-bearing and, parenthetically, whether or not the patient is employing them properly to provide the desired result. During normal gait loads considerably in excess of those provided by simple gravity are borne by the various weight-bearing joints. Let us consider for a moment the loads borne by the hip joint. As the patient stands still on two feet, in the erect position, gravity imposes the weight of the torso above the level of the hips distributed evenly between the two joints during stance. Various muscles are alternately contracting and relaxing to maintain the erect position. As the torso is not perfectly balanced over the hip joints, if all muscles were to simultaneously relax, gravity would quickly topple the unstable elements. Clinically, this is frequently seen in cases of marked muscle weakness, such as muscular dystrophy or poliomyelitis. The purpose of the intermittent contraction of muscles during stance is to counterbalance the pull of gravity. Thus, the more perfectly the center of gravity is aligned over the joint, the less muscle contraction will be required to maintain the erect position. Imagine, however, a patient who is now taking a step or leaning over to pick something off a table or chair. As his center of gravity shifts away from the hip joint, more and more pull must be exerted to keep him from falling. As the mass of his torso moves further away from the center of the joint, there is an increasing magnification of the amount of muscle contraction that must be provided to overcome the pull of gravity, and frequently, even during stance, two to three times the body weight will be imparted to the joint.

Let us consider for a moment how some of these forces act during gait. As we walk, it is apparent that intermittently the hip joint of each lower extremity will be bearing the entire gravitational load of the torso. Now, watch the patient walking from behind. As he steps onto his left foot and lifts the right foot off the ground, the center of gravity falls considerably medial to the center of the hip joint.

19

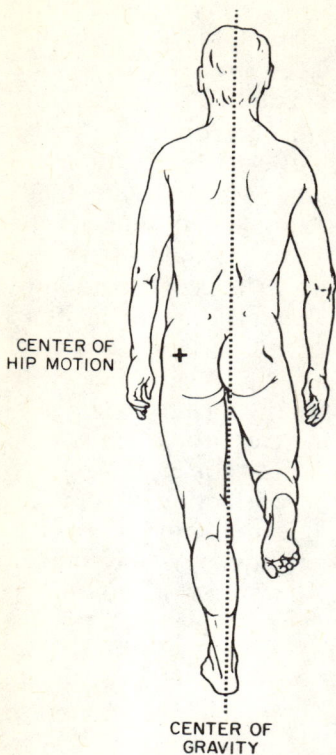

Fig. 6 Center of hip
motion—Frontal Plane

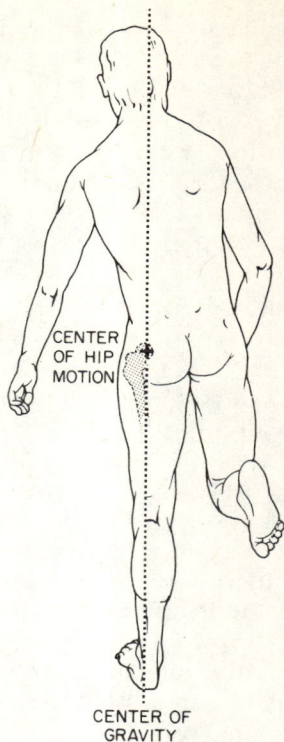

Fig. 7 Balancing center of
hip motion—Frontal Plane

Gravity tends to pull his torso away from his left, weight-bearing extremity. To avoid falling, the patient must do one of two things. He can either counter-balance the pull of gravity by shifting the center of gravity of his torso over the hip or he can counteract the pull of gravity by applying an equal force in the opposite direction. In this instance, an equal force can be applied through the powerful (gluteus medius) abductor mechanism. The application of this force will permit the patient to remain erect and yet allow him to walk without grossly shifting his center of gravity from side to side during alternate steps. The amount of force imparted to the hip joint by the abductor mechanism is roughly equal to the gravitational pull on his torso or body weight.

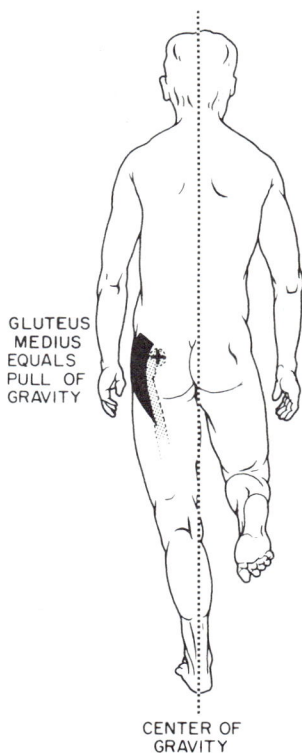

GLUTEUS
MEDIUS
EQUALS
PULL OF
GRAVITY

CENTER OF
GRAVITY

Fig. 8   Compensating center of hip motion—Frontal Plane

In actual practice, during normal gait, both these mechanisms operate and people shift from side to side as they walk, minimizing the amount of force that must be imparted to the hip joint by the abductor mechanism. The next time you are waiting in a line to go to a football game and the line is moving slowly ahead of you, notice how the line constantly undulates from side to side.

21

Now stand to the side of the patient and watch the gait in a lateral plane. As the patient strides forward and bears weight on his right foot, his center of gravity initially is well behind the weight-bearing foot.

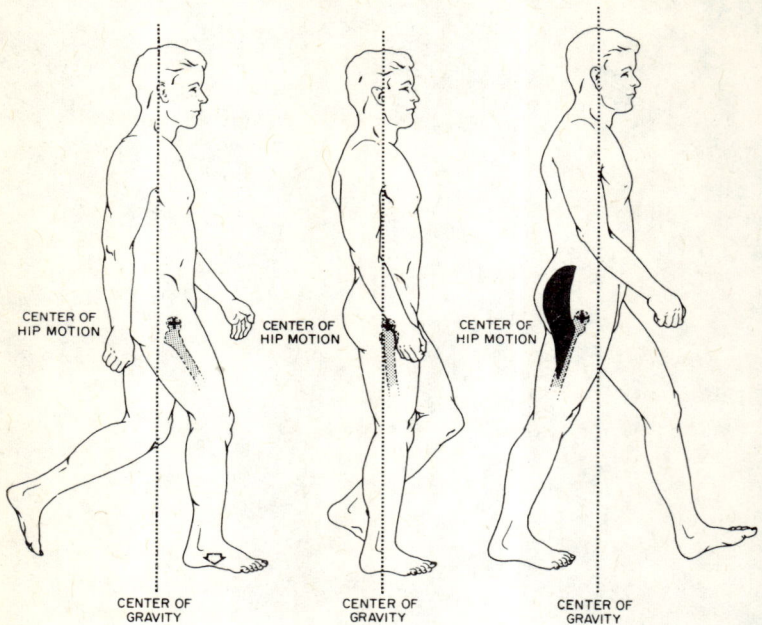

Fig. 9 Center of hip motion —Lateral Plane

Fig. 10 Balancing center of hip motion—Lateral Plane

Fig. 11 Compensating center of hip motion— Lateral Plane

At this point, the weight of his torso tends to topple him over backwards, and it is resisted by contracting his hip (iliopsoas) flexors. As he strides forward, his center of gravity shifts over the hip joint and the force on the hip joint is considerably decreased.

As forward motion continues and the center of gravity passes in front of the weight-bearing right foot, it then tends to topple him forward and this is resisted by the powerful (gluteus maximus) hip extensors until the left foot assumes the weight-bearing load.

The forces imparted to the hip joint by the alternate use of flexors and extensors to maintain the upright position during locomotion are roughly equivalent to balancing the weight of the torso, and thus in the lateral plane muscle contraction also imparts the force of one body weight on the hip joint. Thus, while walking during various phases of locomotion the hip joint assumes a load equal to three body weights (gravity, flexor-extensor balance, and abductor balance).

Now let us see what *canes* and *crutches* do to relieve this. Frequently patients are instructed to walk on crutches to make a joint non-weight-bearing and are asked to carry the affected extremity through a normal range of motion to prevent stiffness during this period of crutch use. Thus, although they relieve the hip joint of the gravitational forces, they continue to impart to it the forces exerted by the muscles acting on the joint. The usual gait employed by a non-weight-bearing patient on crutches is a *"3-point" gait* in which both crutches are placed on the ground simultaneously with the affected limb. This relieves the load of gravity and decreases the amount of muscle input proportionately. However, roughly the equivalent of one body weight is borne by the hip joint due to the muscle activity. Thus, at best, the crutches do not completely relieve weight-bearing on the hip joint, but decreases it from three times body weight to the equivalent of one body weight.

Insofar as the use of a cane is concerned, the usual way of employing it is to have the patient hold the cane in the hand opposite the affected hip, and to transmit load through the cane at the same time that weight is being borne on the affected extremity. Thus, with a painful right

23

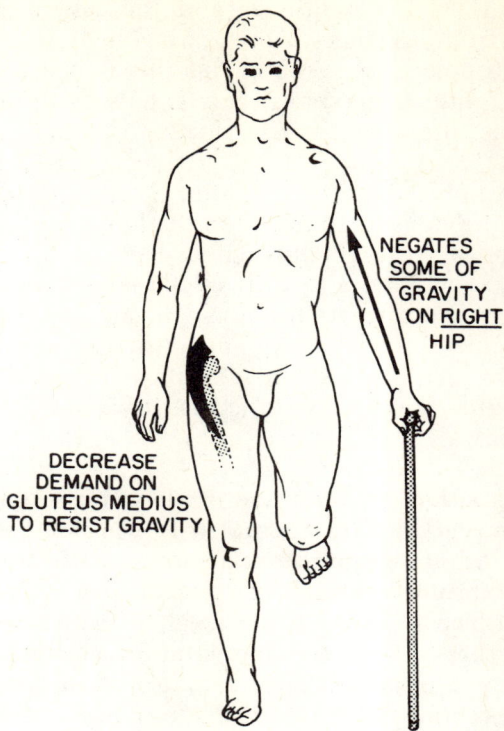

Fig. 12 Relief from a cane—Frontal Plane

hip, the patient is instructed to place the cane in the left hand. As he does so, he accomplishes two things: he decreases the gravitational load on his hip by pushing down with his left hand and with this reduction in gravitational pull, he also decreases the force demanded of the gluteus medius to maintain the erect position. Although this mechanism is not nearly as efficient in relieving weight bearing as the use of crutches, it will relieve roughly the equivalent of one body weight on the hip joint.

In summary, then, we may consider that during normal gait the hip joint bears loads roughly equal to three times body weight, one body weight accounted for by gravity, one body weight accounted for by the abductor mechanism supporting the upright position against the medial pull of gravity, and one body weight accounted for by the flexor-extensor mechanism supporting the upright position against falling either backward or forward, depending upon the phase of gait. The proper use of a cane will subtract roughly one body weight worth of weight-bearing on the hip joint. The proper use of crutches will generally decrease the load on the hip joint by two body weights, but still leaves the equivalent of one body weight of force.

It can be seen that the application of the principles illustrated in the hip joint apply to all of the weight-bearing joints. Thus, in walking up stairs as the right foot is placed on a step, the body weight is propelled upwards by a powerful contraction of the quadriceps to extend the knee and lift the body weight. During this effort, tremendous forces in excess of gravity are placed through the knee joint. When the sprinter runs, as he "pushes off" by powerfully plantar-flexing his foot with the gastrocnemius-soleus complex, forces far in excess of gravitational loads are placed across the ankle joint. When a patient leans over to pick up a newspaper and the center of gravity shifts in front of the spine, forces far in excess of gravitational loads are placed on the spinal joints.

It is evident therefore, that as patients use crutches and canes, they must be observed to get an accurate picture of the effect of these assistive devices and to determine their proper use and effectiveness.

Braces and *casts* are used primarily to provide stability. Casts, being rigid, effectively limit joint motion and provide external stability. Braces, on the other hand, are fabricated in such a way as to provide required stability, but at the same time allow selective joint motion. In the general evaluation of the patient who is using a cast or brace, the effectiveness of the brace or cast should be judged. Since casts are designed to immobilize and restrict joint motion, inquiries should be made of the patient as to whether they can, in fact, move their joints within the cast. Since they are usually used to treat fractures (their function being to provide complete immobilization) inquiries should be made as to whether the patient has a sensation of grating or motion about the fracture site, and whether the cast is effective in relieving pain. Similarly, braces should be evaluated to see that they are meeting the required purpose. This means checking to see if they are properly fitted, that the mechanical joints of the brace are located at the anatomic centers of joint motion, and that they provide the required stability. The purpose of casts and braces are generally apparent to the examiner after he has taken the history, and their effectiveness can be judged during this general part of the examination. Sometimes, however, the requirements of a brace cannot be accurately assessed until a more detailed regional examination of the involved extremity has been conducted. In these instances, the fit of the brace should be judged during the general examination. The brace is then removed for the regional examination, and the effectiveness of the brace is judged again after this more detailed examination.

Many times braces are used not only to provide stability, but also to relieve weight-bearing. In these instances, the examiner should make every effort to determine whether or not the brace is in fact relieving the desired amount of weight. This may be done in various ways. For example, if a brace is fitted to relieve weight from the ankle joint, and transmit it from the shoe to the prepatellar region below the knee, the examiner may slip his finger inside the shoe and ask the patient to stand on the brace to get some estimate of how much weight is actually being transmitted across the ankle joint. While there are more sophisticated methods of making these determinations, in general the effectiveness of braces can be determined by these simple methods.

Let us consider for a moment proper ways in which to describe the findings that have just been discussed. While there is no set method universally employed for each of these various facets of the examination, they should be described in as precise and meaningful terms as possible. Since frequently the examination performed by one physician is used by another, or the initial examination is used as a base-line against which to judge the effectiveness of treatment, general, vague terms are not satisfactory. Thus, to say that the patient walks with a limp on the right is not as meaningful as to say that the patient has antalgic limp with the quick component on the right foot, shifts his center of gravity over the right extremity during weight-bearing and makes facial grimaces indicating discomfort. The description of these physical findings should be done in such a way that your secretary could read them over the phone to a physician in another city and paint a clear picture to that physician of the patient's physical examination.

3. Muscle Power

The evaluation of muscle power is an important diagnostic portion of the musculoskeletal examination. If the patient has no specific complaints relating to weakness or incoordination, muscle power is usually estimated in a general fashion during the early part of the examination; however, if there are specific complaints of weakness or incoordination, a detailed evaluation is done. It is important in this evaluation to describe the power of the muscle in terms of general use so that they may be used later on in comparing the results of treatment or determining the course of a particular process. There are two widely used methods of grading muscle strength. In one system, the muscle is graded numerically beginning at zero for the weakest and ranging through a grade of five. The other system is divided into the same gradations designated by descriptive terms. The six grades are as follows:

a) *Zero or 0.* This describes a situation in which, despite the patient's effort to move a joint with a specific muscle, he can neither produce any motion in the joint, nor can he even produce a palpable contraction for the examiner's hand. When muscles are so weak that they will fall into this category, they must be examined carefully by palpation, and the joint that would be moved by the muscle being examined must be placed in such a fashion that gravity is eliminated. Thus, when testing a patient's very weak quadriceps, to have him sit on the edge of the examining table with the leg hanging down and ask him to extend his knee would make it impossible to differentiate between absolutely no function and very weak function of the quadriceps.

b) *Trace or 1.* This grade describes the muscle that is unable to move the joint, and yet the examiner can feel a palpable contraction.

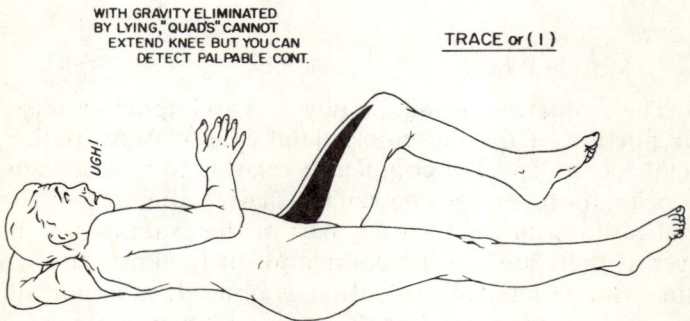

WITH GRAVITY ELIMINATED
BY LYING,"QUADS" CANNOT
EXTEND KNEE BUT YOU CAN
DETECT PALPABLE CONT.

TRACE or (I)

UGH!

Fig. 13 Muscle Grade of Trace (1)

c) *Poor or 2.* In this gradation the muscle being examined can produce motion in the applicable joint, but is unable to produce motion when asked to overcome gravity. It can only do so with gravity eliminated. Thus, the patient whose quadriceps cannot extend the knee in a sitting position, but can do so when lying on the side with gravity eliminated, would have a grade of poor.

28

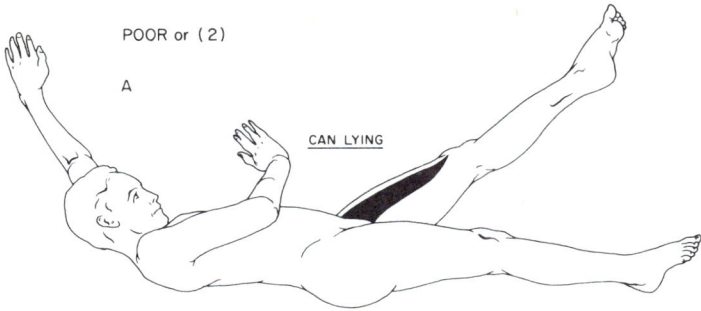

POOR or (2)

A

CAN LYING

A) Recumbent

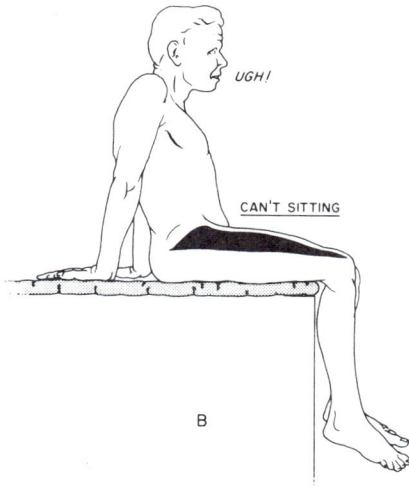

UGH!

CAN'T SITTING

B

B) Sitting

Fig. 14 Muscle Grade of Poor (2)

29

d) *Fair or 3*. This grade of muscle power describes a muscle which can put a joint through a full range of motion against gravity, but is unable to overcome any additional resistance. Thus, the patient who is sitting on the edge of a table and can extend his knee, but who is unable to lift a pound weight with his foot while doing so, would have a grade of fair.

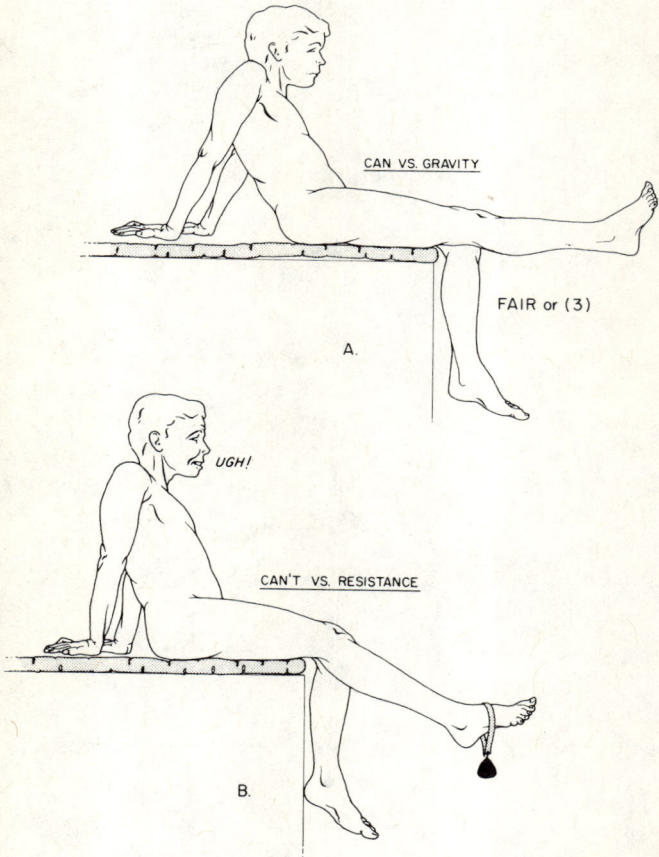

Fig. 15   Muscle Grade of Fair (3)

e) *Good or 4.* A grade of good is assigned to a muscle when it can put the applicable joint through a range of motion and overcome resistance, but is unable to overcome the same amount of resistance that the other unaffected contralateral muscle is able to overcome.

f) *Normal or 5.* This simply describes the ability of a muscle to put a joint through a full range of motion overcoming the normal amount of resistance for a muscle of this particular bulk.

Although this system is a relatively objective system, the subjective skill of the examiner should try to define it further. Thus, grades of plus or minus may be assigned to these descriptive terms. For example, the patient who can completely extend his knee and lift 2 pounds but not 5 pounds would probably be assigned a grade of "fair-plus," while the patient who could lift 15 to 20 pounds would probably be assigned a grade of "good-minus." The strength of individual muscles in these terms, is described as an integral part of the patient's "workup" when his complaint of weakness involves a specific, anatomic, and usually well-localized region. In other situations where the patient may have generalized weakness, such as after a spinal cord injury or paralytic neurologic disease, it is important to examine all muscles carefully and grade them accurately. These grades then are recorded on a special chart in their appropriate terms for each individual muscle.

Accurate compilation of these charts is fundamental to assess the course of a disease or the effect of treatment in these generalized conditions. Since this type of examination has a subjective component to it, it is highly desirable, when the examination is being repeated at intervals, to have it done by the same examiner.

Let us stop now for a moment and consider the various situations in which muscle weakness is commonly seen.

31

1. *Muscle atrophy.* Simple atrophy of disuse is by far and away the most common cause of muscle weakness. This disuse may be secondary to the application of a cast for treatment of a fracture, it may involve the patient's lack of use due to pain in an extremity, or it may be due

UNIVERSITY OF FLORIDA HEALTH CENTER
Department of Physical Therapy
Muscle Examination

Name _____ Age_____ Physician_____
Diagnosis_____ Onset_____

				Therapist	Date				
				Left	Rigt				
Neck &				St. C1-3 Sternocleidomastoid(Acessory St.					
Trunk				Cl. " " Cl.					
				C C1-6 Back Extensore C					
				D T1-T9 " D					
				L T10-15 " L					
				T12-L2 Quadratus Lumborum					
				Ly. C6-8 Latissimus (Thoracodorsal) Ly.					
				Sit. " " " Sit.					
				T7-10 Upper Rectus					
				T10-L1 Lower Rectus					
				T7-10 External Oblique					
				T10-L1 Internal Oblique					
				T7-10 External Oblique					
				T10-L1 Internal Oblique					
Hip				L5-S1 Gluteus Maximus (Inf. Gluteal)					
				L4-S1 Gluteus Medius (Sup. Gluteal)					
				L4-S1 Tensor Fasciae Latae (Sup. Gluteal)					
				L1-4 Iliopsoas					
				L2-4 Sartorius (Femoral)					
				L2-S1 Hip Adductors (Obturator)					
				Lat.L3-S2 Hip Rotators Lat.					
				Med. L4-S2 " Med.					
Knee				L2-4 Quadriceps (Femoral)					
				In. L4-S2 Hamstrings (Sciatic) In.					
				Out. L5-S3 " " Out.					
Foot				Ly. S1-2 Gastrocnemius Soleus (Tibial) Ly.					
				St. " " " St.					
				L4-5 Anterior Tibial (Peroneal)					
				L5-S2 Posterior Tibial (Tibial)					
				L4-5 Peroneals (Peroneal)					
Toes				L4-S1 Extensor Digitorum Longus(Peroneal)					
				L4-S1 Extensor Digitorum Brevis(peroneal)					
				L4-S2 Extensor Hallucis Longus (Peroneal)					
				L5-S2 Flexor Hallucis Longus (Tibial)					
				L5-S2 Flexor Digitorum Longus (Tibial)					
				L5-S1 Flexor Digitorum Brevis(Plantar)					
				L5-S2 Intrinsics (Plantar)					
				L5-S2 Flexor Hallucis Brevis (Plantar)					

Comments:

100%	5	N	Normal	Complete range of motion against gravity with full resistance.
75%	4	G	Good	Complete range of motion against gravity with moderate resistance.
50%	3	F	Fair	Complete range of motion against gravity.
25%	2	P	Poor	Complete range of motion with gravity eliminated.
10%	1	T	Trace	Evidence of slight contractility. No joint motion
0%	0	0	Zero	No evidence of contractility.

Fig. 16 Muscle Grade Record Form

to many other causes. Perhaps one of the most common examples is that seen in the very rapid atrophy of the quadriceps following painful injuries to the knee. Demonstrable atrophy will be reflected in a decreased grade in terms of muscle evaluation, and can also be confirmed by circumferential measurements of the thigh to demonstrate the decreased bulk of the muscle. In general, there is usually good correlation between the muscle grade and changes in the mass of muscles when they are large, bulky muscles, located superficially, and easily measured. It is important when making these circumferential measurements to note carefully, usually by means of a small drawing in the patient's chart, the precise spot in which the measurement was made. The measurement is made at the same spot on the involved and contralateral extremity and the results are recorded next to the drawing. In this way, if one wishes to repeat the measurement at some future time to assess treatment, the measurements will be in the same area and will be comparable.

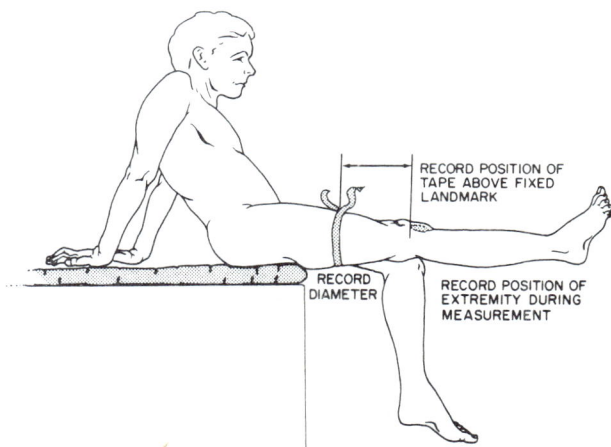

Fig. 17 Circumferential Measurement

A good clinical example might be a boy with a knee injured in football. Following his convalescence, he regains a full range of motion that is painless, but it is important to know that his muscle has regained its full strength prior to letting him resume competitive athletics in order that he may protect his previously damaged knee. Thus, in principle, he should be able to obtain the same muscle grade in this quadriceps as in the uninjured one, and to restore the bulk of the muscle objectively before he will be allowed to play. In addition to grade and bulk, an experienced examiner can gain additional insight into an affected muscle's status by comparing its "tone" to the unaffected side.

2. *Muscle rupture or laceration.* Ruptures of muscles without a penetrating wound or laceration usually occur in one of two situations. In younger people, they occur when the muscle is suddenly loaded beyond its tensile strength. In this situation, the muscle generally fails at the musculotendinous junction. When the patient is asked to contract the muscle, he may not be able to do this without some discomfort but the diagnosis may be somewhat obscure, as the examiner may not know whether this lack is due primarily to mechanical dehiscense or to pain. Careful palpation, revealing a defect, is the most helpful maneuver at this point in time. Later the site of rupture is usually marked by an ecchymosis at an area of localized tenderness. Within a week to 10 days, however, the swelling and edema will subside, the hemorrhage is absorbed and the pain is gone. At this point persistent weakness is accompanied by an increase in the bulk of the muscle just proximal to the site of rupture when the muscle is contracted.

The second clinical setting of a muscle rupture occurs in the older age groups as a result of degenerative changes in the muscle's tendon. These patients may experience rupture frequently under rather minor physiologic loads. Certain muscles are more vulnerable to this by virtue of their mechanical arrangement. These ruptures are generally accompanied by considerably less swelling, tenderness, pain, and ecchymosis than are the traumatic ones in younger individuals. They do, however, present with the same patterns of weakness and the presence of an abnormal bulge.

34

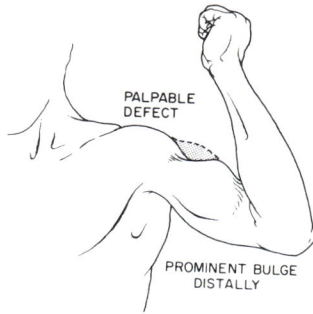

PALPABLE
DEFECT

PROMINENT BULGE
DISTALLY

Fig. 18   Ruptured Biceps

3. *Spastic paralysis.* Decreased muscle grades are frequently encountered with patients who have lost the
reflex smooth coordinate mechanism of muscle contraction. This is generally seen with any upper motor
neuron lesion which leaves the spinal reflex arc intact but
deprives the neural complex of inhibitory and facilitory
impulses to coordinate these activities. On examination,
these muscles feel tight and tense as if the patient were
already contracting them. Yet when they are asked to produce motion or overcome loads they are considerably
weaker than a normal muscle would be. The reflexes that
accompany this kind of muscle activity are both hyperac-
tive and in many instance, pathologic. This type of muscle
weakness is typically seen in the child with cerebral palsy.
It is just as important to grade the function of muscles in
this patient, as it is in patients with the more classical spastic paralysis due to a stroke. These patients generally do
not complain of weakness, but more likely of incoordinate
movement. Frequently their lack of coordination represents not only their neurologic disease, but differential
grades of strength between various antagonistic sets of
muscles. Thus, they may have strong flexors of the forearm
and weak extensors, and this imbalance may produce a
flexion contracture of the wrist. Since surgical procedures
are frequently done on such patients to correct deformities
by relieving the spastic muscles, it is important to grade

35

their strength before attempting such releases to assure that the remaining function will be adequate to carry out tasks within the patient's ability.

4. *Flaccid paralysis.* These muscles are just the opposite of spastic muscles. They are small, atrophic, flabby, and weak with decreased reflexes. They too may be accompanied by deformities, but in this instance, the deforming force is the unparalyzed or normal muscle which overcomes the paralyzed, weakened muscle. The patient who has had flaccid paralysis of the dorsiflexors of the foot with a normal gastrocnemius, will frequently show a fixed equinus deformity due to the imbalance.

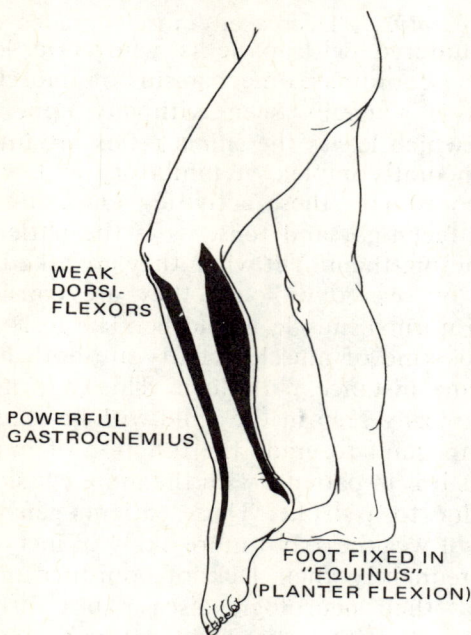

WEAK
DORSI-
FLEXORS

POWERFUL
GASTROCNEMIUS

FOOT FIXED IN
"EQUINUS"
(PLANTER FLEXION)

Fig. 19 Deformity due to Muscle Imbalance

Frequently, these deformities, or loss of function due to flaccid paralysis may be partially or completely restored by a *muscle transfer* to replace lost function. When the mus-

36

cle is transferred, it is important to evaluate its strength (grade) prior to transfer. As a principle, one must figure that a transposed muscle will function a grade weaker than it will in its normal position. A clinical example of such a situation would be the child who has a femoral nerve palsy resulting in complete paralysis of the quadriceps muscles in the thigh. As a result, this child frequently will fall when trying to walk because of the inability to stabilize the knee in extension while bearing weight. In order to ambulate satisfactorily, the child will have to wear a long leg brace with a locking device at the knee to prevent this inadvertent buckling or giving-way when bearing weight. Another way of treating this would be to transfer the flexors (hamstrings) from behind the knee and reroute them to insert in the patella to substitute for the paralyzed quadriceps. In order to function satisfactorily so that the patient may be relieved of the brace (which is the purpose of the operation) the patient will have to use the transposed muscle to stabilize the knee when walking uphill. This requires a grade of "fair-plus" or "good-minus" in the transposed hamstring. In turn, to be available as a motor for the pro-

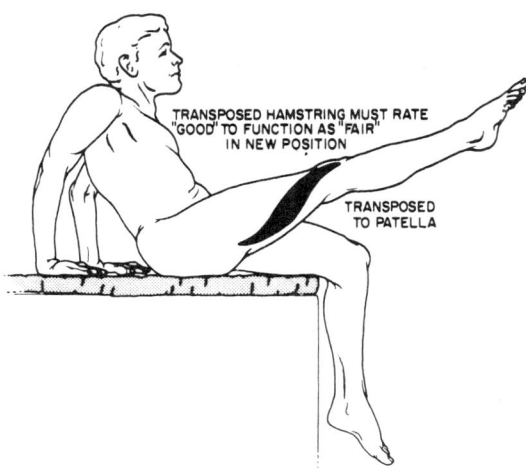

TRANSPOSED HAMSTRING MUST RATE "GOOD" TO FUNCTION AS "FAIR" IN NEW POSITION

TRANSPOSED TO PATELLA

Fig. 20   Muscle Transfer

posed operation, the hamstring in its normal position must have a rating of "good-plus" or "normal-minus." It is obvious that if the hamstring in its normal position rates only "good-minus" and loses a grade in the course of the transfer, it will end up functioning at a fair-minus level in the transposed position. The patient will be able to extend the knee with gravity eliminated, but will be unable to walk without the use of a brace, and thus will have had an ineffective operation.

4. Joint Motion

Frequently, in examining the musculoskeletal system, measurements of ranges of joint motion are made. It is important to describe these in the patient's record accurately for purposes of assessing the results of treatment or following the course of diseases, or as a reference point if changes occur. Such statements as "the patient lacks 45° of extension and the last 40° of flexion" or "he has a range of motion from 45° of flexion to 80° of flexion" are accurately descriptive as opposed to "his motion is limited." The following descriptions and examples of measurements illustrate some of the terminology used and some of the methods and applications of these kinds of examination. Although they are applicable to all regions of the body, they are used more commonly in some regions than others and will be again commented on in the portions of the text, devoted to regions.

In describing joint motion, one must specify whether the *motion is active or passive.* Active means that the patient is able to perform it himself by the use of his muscles, while passive describes the motion produced by the examiner. Many times it is important to measure both the active and passive ranges of motion in the particular joint. For example, in the patient who comes in stating that he is unable "to straighten out my knee," this lack of motion might be due to either weakness of the quadriceps mechanism or an internal mechanical block of motion in the joint. If the patient is examined in a sitting position and can actively extend the knee only to minus 15°, but the examiner can passively extend it completely to 0°, it would be apparent that the cause was muscle weakness.

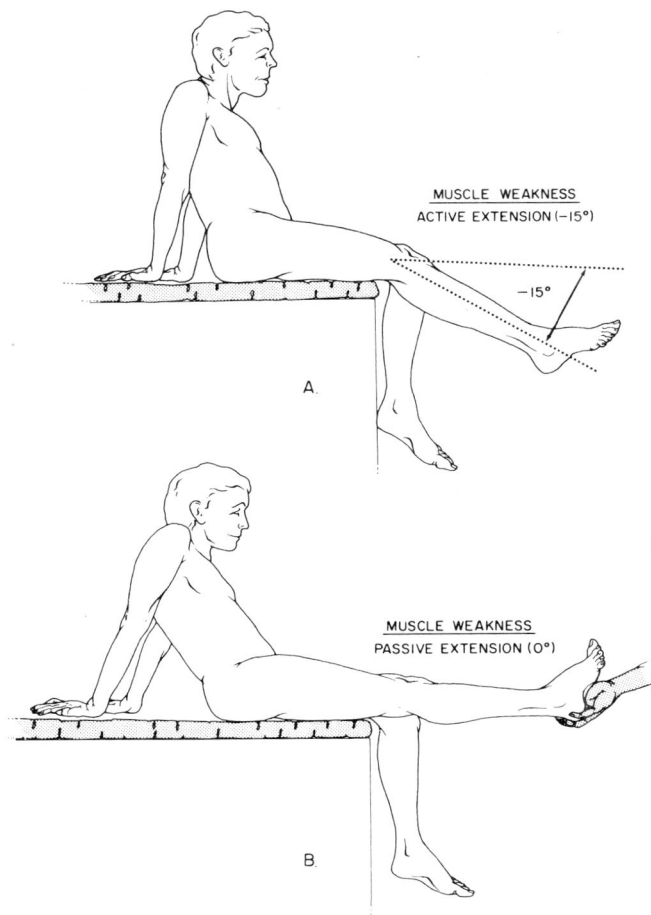

MUSCLE WEAKNESS
ACTIVE EXTENSION (−15°)

−15°

A.

MUSCLE WEAKNESS
PASSIVE EXTENSION (0°)

B.

Fig. 21   Interpretations of Active and Passive Motion

39

However, if the patient could only actively extend it to minus 15° and the examiner could only passively extend it to the same range of motion, and could feel good, strong, palpable contraction of the patient's quadriceps, it would turn attention to internal derangement of the knee as the cause.

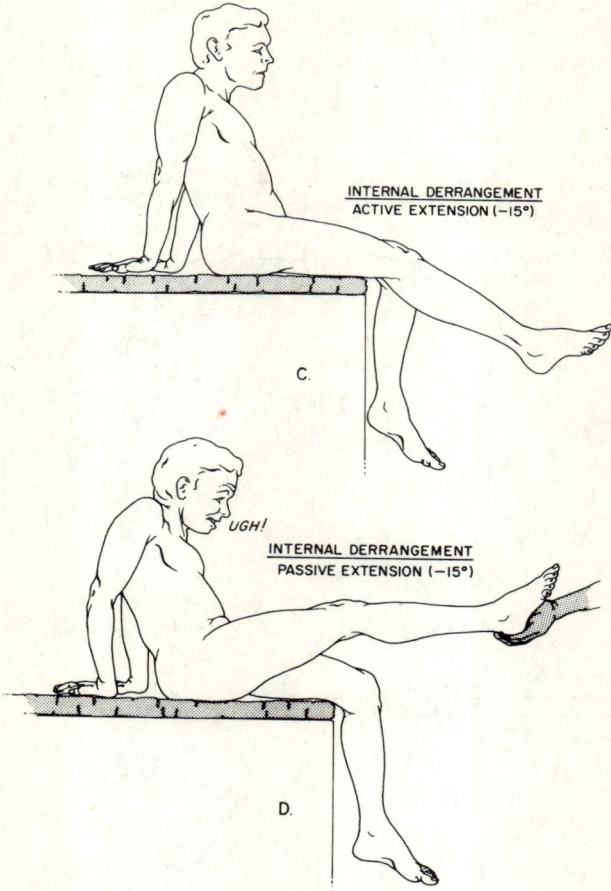

INTERNAL DERRANGEMENT
ACTIVE EXTENSION (−15°)

C.

UGH!

INTERNAL DERRANGEMENT
PASSIVE EXTENSION (−15°)

D.

Fig. 21   Interpretations of Active and Passive Motion

40

In describing joint motion, it is important to describe the plane through which the motion is taking place. There are six such planes of motion, and they are determined by their relationship to the midline of the body or the extremity.

1. *Flexion.* Meaning to bend. In flexion, the portion of the joint moved is brought toward the midline when viewed in the saggital or lateral plane.

2. *Extension.* Meaning to straighten. This is the reverse of flexion. In this motion, the portion of the limb being moved is carried away from the midplane of the body.

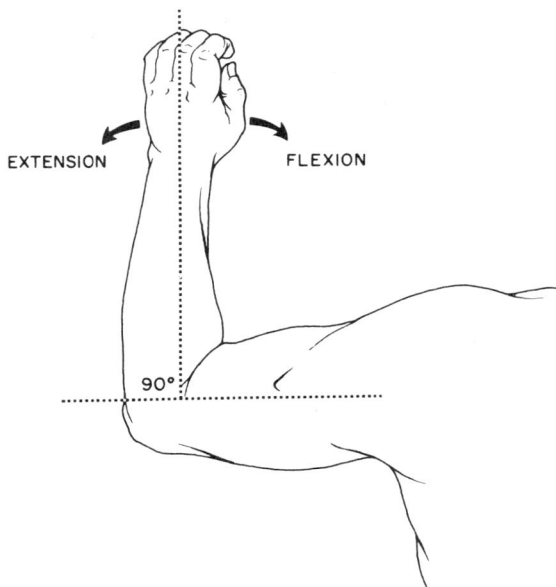

Fig. 22   Flexion — Extension

3. *Abduction.* Meaning to take away. In this plane of motion, the extremity being moved is carried away from the midline when viewed in the coronal or frontal plane.

4. *Adduction.* Meaning to bring toward. This is motion toward the midline of the body.

41

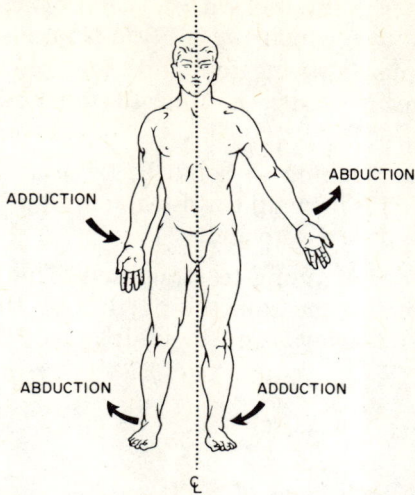

Fig. 23 Abduction — Adduction

5. *Internal rotation.* Meaning to twist toward. This is rotary motion in which the extremity rotates in the plane of the cross section of the body toward the midline.

6. *External rotation.* Meaning to twist away. This is rotary motion in the transverse plane away from the midline.

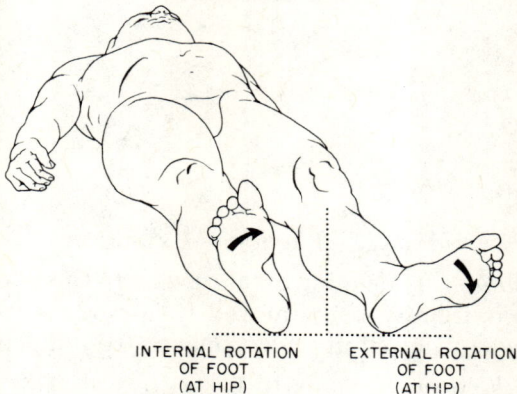

INTERNAL ROTATION
OF FOOT
(AT HIP)

EXTERNAL ROTATION
OF FOOT
(AT HIP)

Fig. 24 Internal — External Rotation

Since many joints are able to carry out all of these ranges of motion, they may be combined in various degrees to produce circumduction. These are the ball-and-socket joints such as the hip or shoulder. Other joints, such as the knee, ankle, and elbow by virtue of the stability which they must have, are essentially one-plane joints (flexion and extension). Other motions which would make them unstable are prevented by bony anatomy or ligamentous structures.

In describing these motions, they are expressed in degrees as a range of motion (ROM). In expressing the ranges of motion, the neutral or zero-degree position is the position one assumes when standing at military attention. Thus, complete extension of the elbow is zero degrees, and the range of motion of the elbow would be described as from 0-120° of flexion, meaning that the patient was able to carry the forearm from a fully extended position to a position of 120° of flexion. In the various regional parts of the text, normal ranges of motion for those particular joints will be described in more detail.

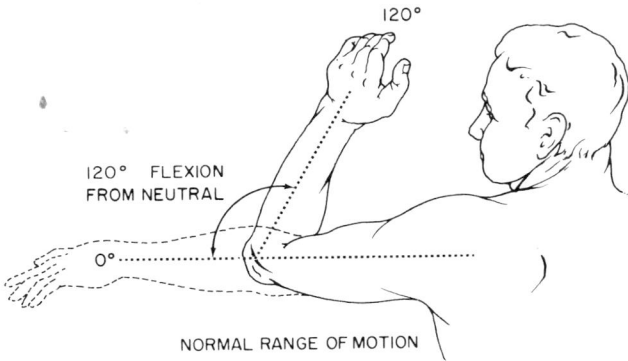

120°

120° FLEXION
FROM NEUTRAL

0°

NORMAL RANGE OF MOTION

Fig. 25   Range of Elbow Motion

Lack of a normal range of motion is described as limitation of either active or passive motion in degrees. It is well to qualify normal ranges of motion with an appropriate

43

explanatory description. Thus, the statement "the patient is unable to extend the knee actively and lacks the last 10° of extension. When passive extension is tested it appears to reach an abrupt, firm stop," is more descriptive than simply stating "the last 10° of extension is missing." It is also well to try to interpret these alterations in ranges of motion in view of the patient's chief complaint and general findings. Thus, the statement that "the patient lacks 10° of active extension accounting for the limp and painful left leg" might be appropriate.

Again in examining joints, abnormal motion representing instability should be accurately described. If the patient has had, for example, a tear of the collateral ligament allowing a valgus deformity of the knee and instability on examination, this is better recorded by a statement such as "the patient has a mild/moderate/severe degree of medial instability on forced abduction" rather than "the patient's knee is unstable."

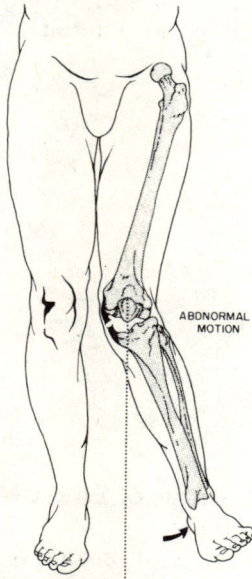

Fig. 26   Joint Instability

44

5. Limb Length and Girth

Limb lengths are measured most commonly with a tape measure from fixed bony landmarks, but under certain circumstances, x-ray measurements are used. If one tries to compare the lengths of the lower extremities by observing the position of the feet in the supine position one may be misled by *"functional shortening"* as opposed to *"true shortening"* of an extremity. Functional shortening of an extremity generally comes about because the patient has a fixed adduction contracture of the hip joint. With the hip joint fixed in 30° or more of adduction, in order to keep the extremities uncrossed for function, the patient will lift the pelvis on the affected side. By doing so, the limbs can be uncrossed even though the fixed adduction contracture is not overcome. When the limbs are uncrossed, however, there appears to be a marked difference in the lengths of the lower extremities. The amount of this difference is equal to the amount the pelvis has been raised above the horizontal.

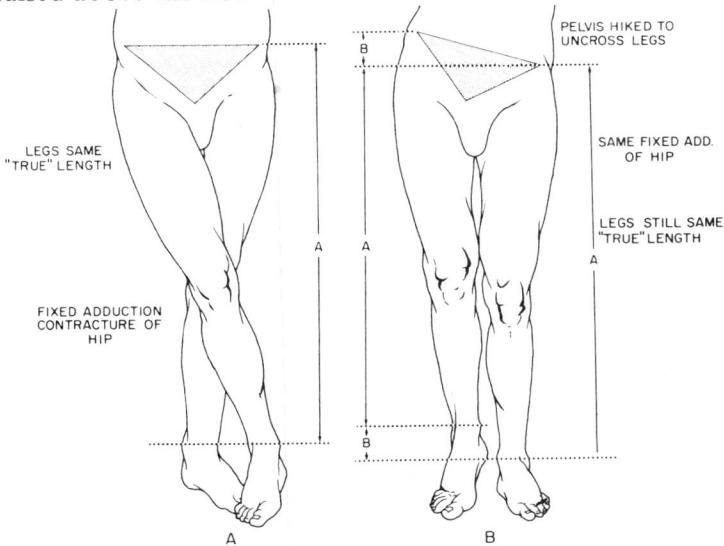

Fig. 27 Functional Shortening

45

In order to determine, then, if shortening of the lower extremity is due to a functional position of the hip or to true shortening, the measurements are made from fixed bony landmarks. The commonly used landmarks for the lower extremity are the anterior superior iliac spine to the medial malleolus with the hip, knee, and ankle in neutral alignment. Figure 28 demonstrates the common landmarks used for various anatomic regions.

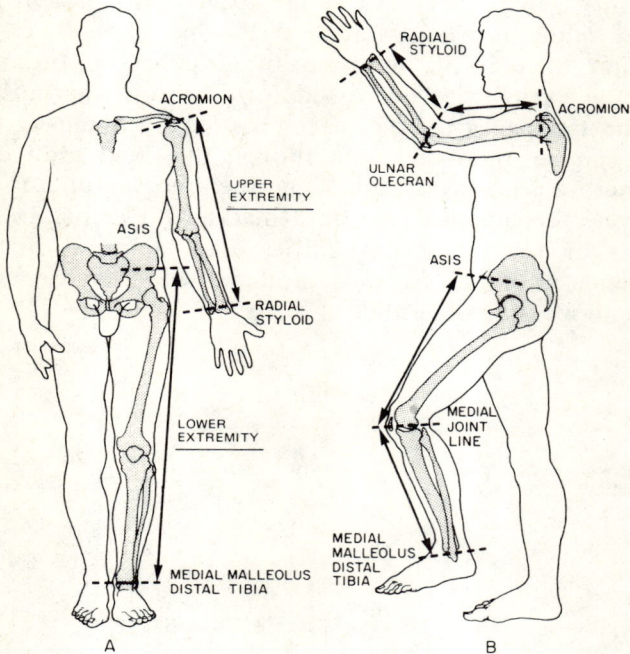

Fig. 28 Common skeletal landmarks A) Frontal B) Lateral

In children with significant growth remaining, inequality in length of the extremities, particularly the lower extremities, is a common therapeutic problem. In a growing child a significantly shortened extremity may be corrected in one of three ways. 1) It may be attacked directly by surgical procedures that lengthen the shortened leg. The

46

effectiveness of these procedures, however, is limited by the amount of stretch one can safely put on vessels and nerves and the bony gap that one can get to heal. This is generally limited to about 5 cm. 2) The second method is to wait until the child has completed his growth and compensate for the inequality by either builtup shoes or by surgical procedures to remove length from the longer extremity. This is not very commonly done. 3) A third method, and perhaps the most commonly used, is to estimate the amount of growth remaining and prematurely surgically close the epiphyseal growth plates in the longer extremity. Closure is done at a time when anticipated growth of the shorter extremity will equalize limb length by the time growth is complete. A method of accurately estimating the amount of subsequent growth that will occur in the given extremity over a given period of time is required. Such tables have been prepared and are available.

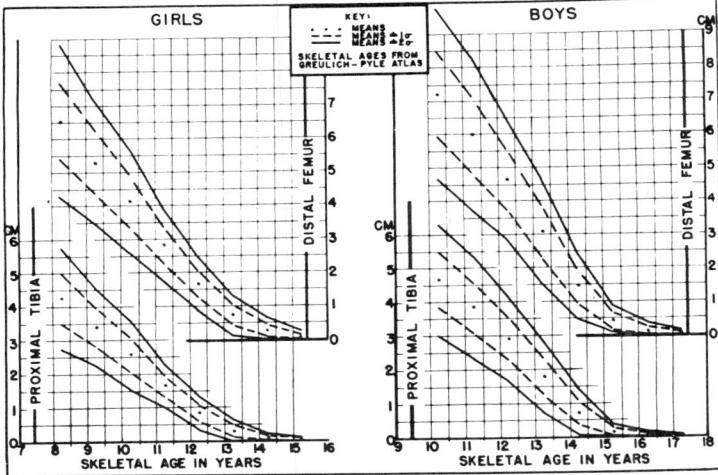

Fig. 29   Predictive Growth Chart (Anderson-Green)

Looking at the table one sees that there are different rates for boys and girls and so two tables are available. One simply looks at the side of the tables and selects the amount of shortening to be compensated and follows this line across horizontally until it intersects the growth curve and then drops vertically to the bottom to obtain the age at which a closure of a normal epiphysis will gain the desired equalization. By selecting the proper time and/or the proper epiphysis, one can forecast this with accuracy of .5 cm. It is well to note that there is a fairly wide range around the median and if the patient in question is a rapidly growing child with tall parents, the upper portions of the range should be used and the lower portions of the range for contrasting children. One can also, knowing the age of the child, predict with some accuracy the growth remaining by using the table in the reverse fashion.

In using growth tables, it is well to realize that years represent not the chronological age of the child, but his skeletal maturation in years. Accurate determination of the maturation of the skeleton can only be told by x-ray examination. One way of doing this is to x-ray regions of certain epiphyses to see whether or not they have appeared. Since the time of the appearance of many epiphyses is rather constant, this gives an accurate check as to whether the child's skeletal maturity matches his chronological age. A chart displaying the appearance of the shafts and the various secondary ossification centers (epiphyses) and the time of closure of the various epiphyseal plates is shown in the appendix.

Even more precise estimates of skeletal age can be made by studying x-rays of the wrist and hand for the appearance of the epiphyseal plates and the ossification centers about the hand. Thus, the radiograph of a child can be compared with the standard radiologic appearance at time intervals of six months. (Gruenlich and Pyle, *et al*), and one can then determine with a good deal of accuracy the patient's skeletal age within six months. It is this skeletal age that is used in estimating growth from the growth charts. One can see from the chart that in accuracy of within six months insofar as skeletal age is concerned is sufficient.

When clinical problems require estimates of growth and operative procedures are based on these estimates, it is necessary to measure length in a more accurate fashion than can be done clinically from bony landmarks. This is generally done by x-ray examination, by a procedure most commonly called a *"scanogram."* In this examination, the patient lies on an x-ray cassette (film holder) that has a linear metal scale which will be transmitted to the x-ray film when the x-ray is exposed. The tube of the x-ray machine is centered over the proximal end of the limb and half of the film exposed. The tube is next centered over the distal area to be measured and the other half of the film is exposed. This does not give an overall x-ray of the bone to be measured as ordinary technique magnifies the size of the bone on the x-ray by approximately 25%. However, by centering the tube over the proximal and distal ends and superimposing the image on the linear scale, the magnification effect is cancelled and one can simply measure on the x-ray the corresponding areas for true measurements. This type of examination is done periodically to accurately assess changes during growth.

Methods of measuring muscle mass circumferentially at a measured distance from a fixed bony landmark have already been discussed. It is important when noting changes in size due to deformities or abnormal masses to record their location with respect to fixed bony landmarks accurately. One of the better ways of doing this is to make a rough sketch in the patient's chart, filling in the measurements in the most appropriate manner. If one is trying to estimate whether a given mass is enlarging or not, he needs to observe it over a period of time to see what happens to it and in this instance, such measurements become crucial. A more accurate way of doing this is to palpate the outlines of the mass, mark them with a skin pencil, and then

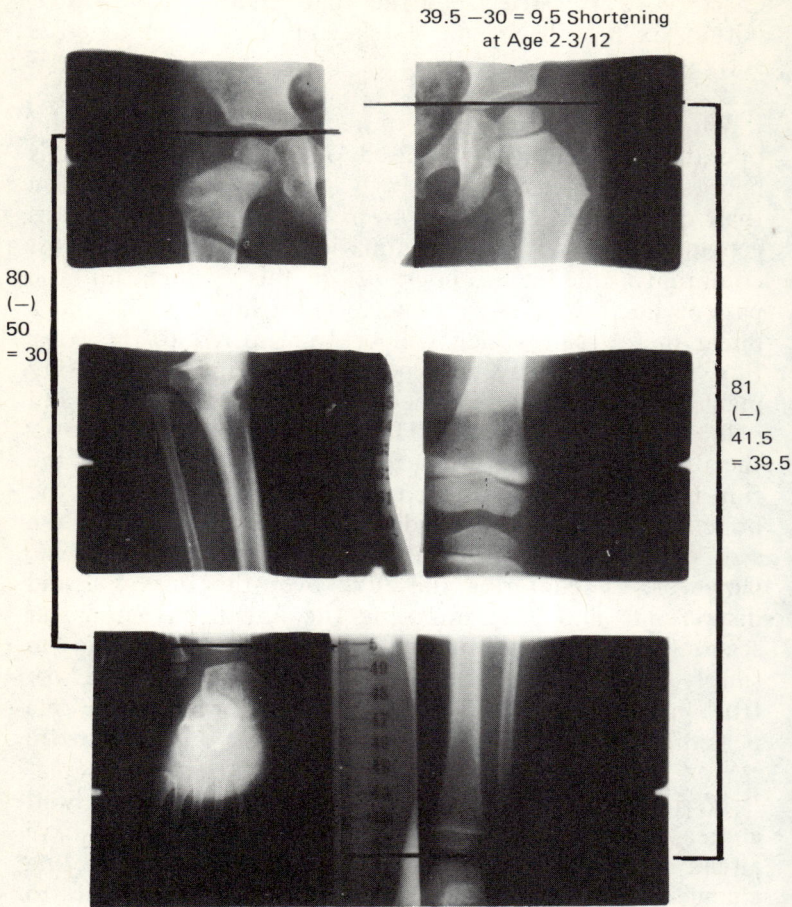

Fig. 30 Scanogram

photograph the region. Whatever method is used, however, it is important to record the method of determination accurately, so that when measurements are redone at a later interval, they do not give a false impression because they have been done in a different way.

6. Physical Manifestations of Trauma

Since many of the patients who present themselves for orthopaedic care and consultation do so because of injuries, it is well to be aware of the various physical signs and the methods of examination following *acute trauma.* This is particularly true when there is no superficial change on visual inspection.

The most common physical finding following injury is swelling. At first edema is soft, usually compressable, and begins to appear within 15-30 minutes following the injury. As soon as it is appreciated in an injured extremity and the examination of the extremity has been completed, the continued swelling should be treated by the application of gentle continuous external pressure. This is usually most effectively done by the use of air splints or carefully applied elastic bandages.

The presence of subcutaneous bleeding in the absence of a laceration, the common "black-and-blue" marks, denote hemorrhage deep within the tissues. Such ecchymoses either may appear fairly rapidly or may not appear for as long as 48 hours, depending on the depth of the bleeding. When present, however, in the swollen extremity with localized tenderness, an ecchymosis is usually suggestive of a fracture or some major tissue damage. When intra-articular hemorrhage occurs, it usually denotes significant tearing of intra-articular structures. Frequently a hemarthrosis will not become apparent externally for several days because the hemorrhage must dissect from the damaged joint to the subcutaneous tissues. The speed at which swelling of a joint increases helps to distinguish between bleeding (rapid) and reactive synovial effusion (slow). If in doubt, aspiration of the joint will settle the question.

In the presence of swelling and ecchymosis when the patient is first examined, the extremity should be carefully examined for instability. This examination must be done gently in a way that is as painless as possible to the patient.

If one is able to show instability, meaning either a significant ligament rupture or a fracture in the extremity, do not carry the limb to the limits of instability at the initial examination. Identifying the instability is the important issue at this point. When one is examining such an injured extremity, he must examine carefully every bone and every joint in the extremity for instability rather than attempt to examine the extremity as a whole. When instability is present, as soon as the examination is completed, the extremity should be splinted until definitive care can be rendered. This splinting by prepared or homemade apparatus, as the occasion warrants, is not only for the patient's comfort, but also to immobilize fractures. This prevents further damage to soft tissues, and the inadvertent penetration of the bone ends through the skin, and reduces muscle spasm which occurs involuntarily when there is instability and may handicap subsequent treatment.

If one has found an area of instability in a swollen ecchymotic extremity, he should examine it very carefully to see whether he may elicit crepitation. Crepitation is the term used to denote the sensation one feels through his hands or hears when two ends of a fracture move against each other. This has been likened to the sound of loose gravel, but it really must be felt and heard to be appreciated. Crepitation, of course, indicates that a fracture is present and requires immediate splinting.

After a swollen, ecchymotic, unstable extremity with localized crepitation has been examined and before splinting is done, both the neurologic and circulatory status of the extremity should be quickly determined. This is done not only to find out whether the structures such as the major arteries and nerves have been damaged by the injury, but also as a guide in future management. For example, suppose that a patient has been admitted to the hospital with a fracture dislocation of the ankle with a marked deformity, and an inexperienced physician sees him, notes the deformity, and orders an x-ray which reveals the precise extent of the injury. A general anesthetic is then administered and the injury is reduced by manipulation. After reduction, subsequent examination reveals that the dorsalis pedis pulse is absent. At this time, the physician is faced with the question, was the circulation destroyed by the initial injury and reduction failed to restore it, or was it present and the reduction in fact caused the circulatory loss. Such an example points out the importance of checking the circulation prior to the initial splinting.

Another example might be the patient admitted following an automobile accident with an obvious posterior dislocation of the hip which is quickly confirmed by x-ray and a closed reduction achieved. Following the reduction, however, the patient is unable to dorsiflex his foot and has a sensory loss consistent with a complete loss of function over the peroneal branch of the sciatic nerve. Was this caused by the original dislocation, or has the nerve been damaged in the course of the reduction? What now should be done to relieve it? Again, a prereduction examination would have solved this distressing problem.

The principles of managing patients with injuries will be discussed later on in the text, but it is probably well at this point to define the terms by which fractures and/or dislocations are usually described. Proper use of these terms should enable the physician to describe the fracture over the telephone to another physician enabling him to accurately reproduce the clinical picture.

1. *Fracture.* Any disruption in the continuity of a bone.

2. *Dislocation. (Luxation).* A disruption in the continuity of a joint. Fractures are never dislocated; they may be displaced, but never dislocated. The two may occur together. That is, there may be a fracture of one of the bones forming the joint and a concomitant dislocation, in which case there is said to be a fracture-dislocation.

3. *Subluxation.* A disruption in the continuity of a joint but without complete dislocation. A synonym might be an incomplete dislocation.

4. *Closed (simple) Fracture.* This is a fracture in which the bones have not penetrated the overlying skin or overlying lacerations do not reach the bone. This term is used in contrast to open (compound).

5. *Open (compound) Fracture.* An open fracture or dislocation is one in which the bone or joint communicates freely with the external air. It may have been opened from within by the bone penetrating the overlying skin to the air, or it may have been opened by a laceration communicating with the fracture site.

6. *Comminuted.* This term is used in describing fractures and indicates that there are more than two fragments at the fracture site. If there are multiple fragments, the fracture may be said to be severely comminuted.

7. *Greenstick Fracture.* A term applied to fractures in children in which the x-ray appearance suggests that one-half of the cortex of the bone remains intact while the other half is fractured. In truth, the fracture line of these injuries extends all the way across the bone, but a tough hinge of periosteum keeps them from displacing. Indeed, they do have the appearance of a bent green twig.

After having applied these terms to a fracture, the amount of displacement present is noted as well as the angulation or direction of the fracture line. Thus, the tibial fracture depicted in Figure 31 would be best described as an open fracture of the midshaft of the tibia splinted with an air splint (zipper). The fracture is comminuted. The tibia is bowed posteriorly 10° and the major distal fragment is posteriorly displaced 2 cm. from the major proximal fragment. By thus adding the location and direction to the other descriptive terms, a verbal picture is painted that describes a fracture accurately. This is certainly to be preferred to recording simply that the patient had a "broken leg."

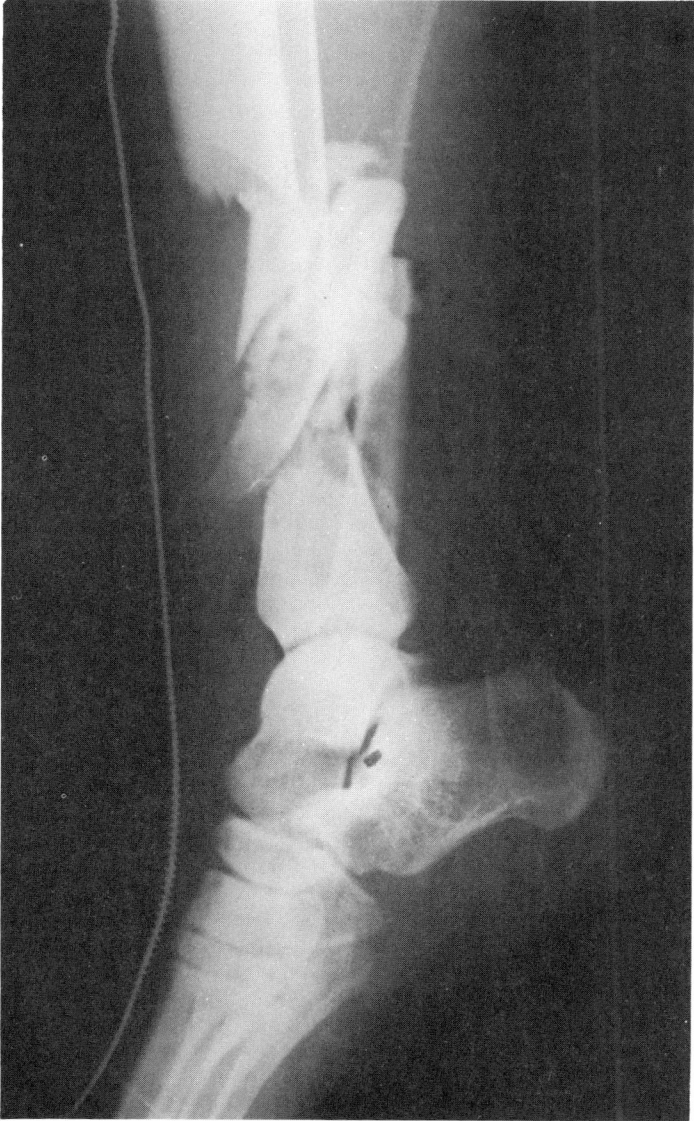

Fig. 31 Fracture of the Tibia

B. REGIONAL ORTHOPAEDIC EXAMINATION

In this section the anatomic basis for the physical examination of the major regions of the musculoskeletal system will be presented. In each section the ranges of motion of the joints and how to determine them are demonstrated. The basis of these Figures is the booklet on Joint Motion published by the American Academy of Orthopaedic Surgeons in 1965. The average range of motion for each joint is shown in the appendix of this manual on pages 199 and 200.

1. Foot

Viewed from the bottom the foot is a triangular shaped base that maintains the balance of the body in the upright position. The apex of the triangle is the heel and the base is the heads of the metatarsals.

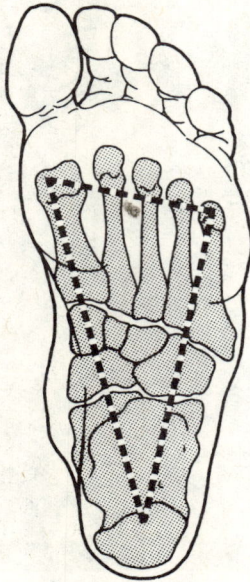

Fig. 32 Weight-Bearing Base of the foot—Plantar Aspect

A normal gait is referred to as a heel-toe gait. The heel strikes first and takes all the weight. Thus the os calcis is covered with a thick fat pad and the overlying skin has highly developed proprioceptive end organs. With locomotion the weight is transferred to the heads of the metatarsals for the push-off portion of the stride.

The sole of the foot should be inspected for any scars or callosities. A foot with a fixed deformity usually will have a painful *callus* over an abnormal bony prominence. In chronic rheumatoid arthritis, callosities frequently occur beneath the heads of all the metatarsals. These are tender to direct palpation. Presence of a callus may also indicate an underlying plantar wart. The *plantar wart* is identified by being tender when the callus is pinched as well as when direct pressure is applied. The presence of the normal cornified skin on the plantar surface of the foot indicates whether the patient is bearing weight and also the distribution of the weight-bearing.

Viewed from the medial side, the normal foot has a *longitudinal arch* that is maintained by the bony configuration of the foot, the long plantar ligaments, the plantar aponeurosis, and the balance of the intrinsic and extrinsic muscles. The foot may be divided into the *forefoot* (toes and metatarsals), *Mid-foot* (tarsals), and the *hind-foot* (talus and calcaneus).

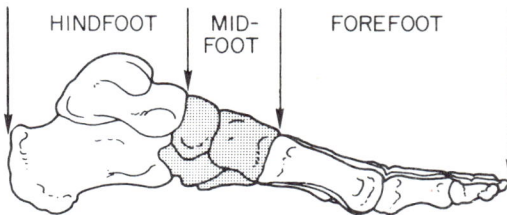

Fig. 33 Medial View of the Foot

57

The general examination of the foot begins by observing the patient standing barefoot on a hard surface. One should observe the presence of hair on the foot, any evidence of discoloration, as well as any gross deformities. Particularly in older patients, hair over the dorsum of the toes is a good index to the circulatory status, i.e., with functional circulatory loss, there is a corresponding diminution in hair. While standing, there is usually an obvious longitudinal arch and the pulps of the toes should touch the floor. Some time in the course of the examination, the foot should be examined for the presence of pulses and for sensation as well as muscle testing. The latter is grossly identified by the patient's ability to walk on his heels and then on his toes. Should the patient be unable to stand with his heel on the floor, he may have an equinus deformity. *Equinus* of the foot is a fixed plantar flexion contracture due to shortening of the posterior structures. The most common causes are cerebral palsy and a portion of the talipes equino-varus (clubfoot) deformity.

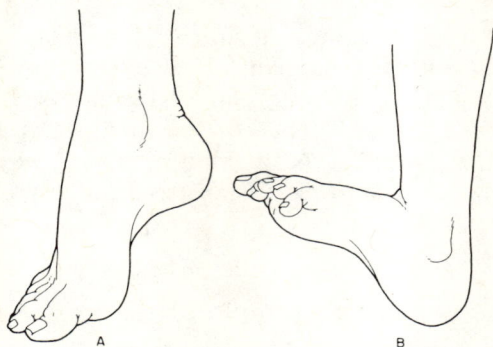

Fig. 34   (A) Equinus and (B) Calcaneal Deformities

The opposite deformity is termed a *"calcaneus"* foot in which the heel is dropped and overly prominent while the longitudinal arch is relatively normal. It is associated with weakness and/or lengthening of the posterior structures usually seen as an insignificant common positional deformity in the newborn which spontaneously corrects.

58

Observation of the arches will indicate the presence or absence of the longitudinal arch. Absence of the longitudinal arch is referred to as *pes planus*. Pes planus is usually congenital or due to muscle paralysis.

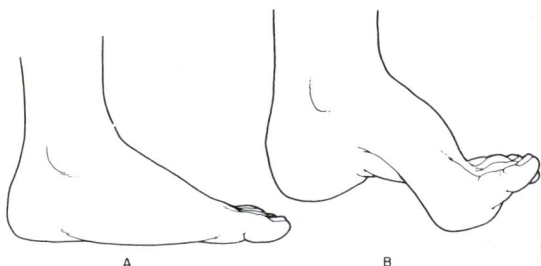

Fig. 35   (A) Pes Planus and (B) Pes Cavus

The contrasting deformity is termed *pes cavus* in which the longitudinal arch is abnormally high. This deformity is most commonly seen with neurologic diseases producing muscle imbalance. It is also frequently combined with other deformities (heel varus and claw toes) in children with meningomyelocele.

If the forefoot is actually dorsiflexed on the hindfoot, the foot appears as a *rocker bottom foot*. This may be referred to as a broken midfoot. The cause of this latter deformity may be an incorrect treatment of talipes equinovarus (clubfoot), or the structural abnormality of the foot known as *congenital convex pes valgus.*

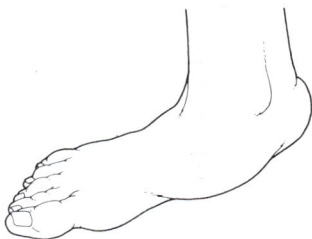

**Fig. 36
Rockerbottom Foot**

Viewed from above the foot is aligned through the ankle with the leg. It moves in a rotary fashion in inversion and eversion and in the frontal plane in abduction and adduction.

59

FORE PART of the FOOT

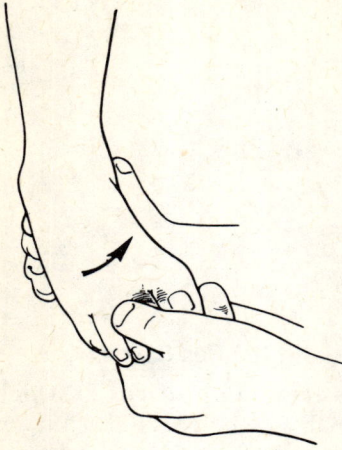

Fig. A INVERSION

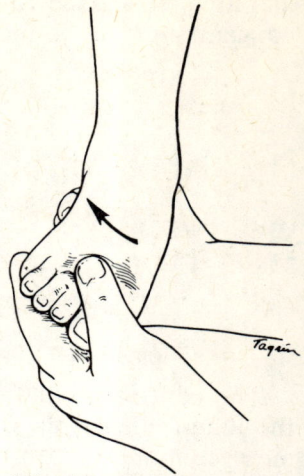

Fig. B EVERSION

Fig. C
PASSIVE ADDUCTION
and ABDUCTION

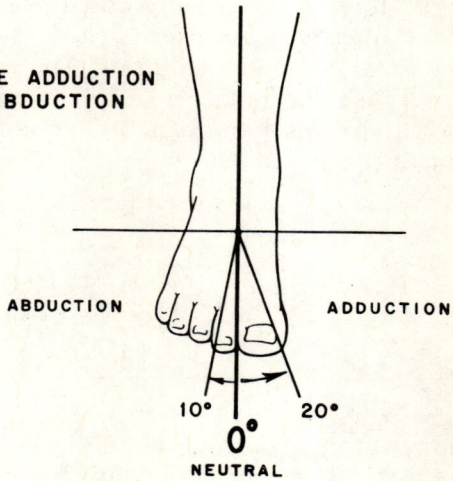

ABDUCTION

ADDUCTION

10°   20°

0°
NEUTRAL

Fig. 37 Motions of the Forefoot

FORE PART of the FOOT

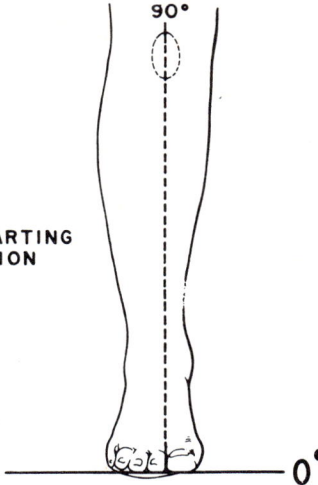

Fig. A
ZERO STARTING
POSITION

90°

0°

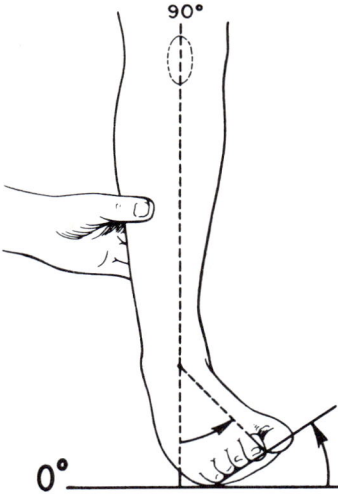

90°

0°

Fig. B INVERSION
$\left(\begin{array}{l}\text{SUPINATION, ADDUCTION}\\\text{AND PLANTAR FLEXION}\end{array}\right)$

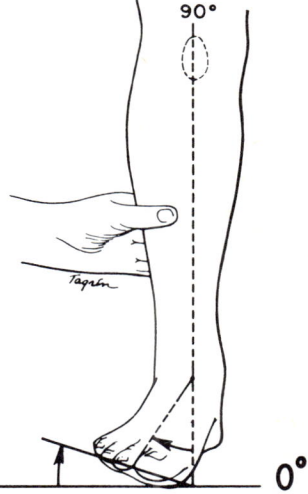

90°

0°

Fig. C EVERSION
$\left(\begin{array}{l}\text{PRONATION, ABDUCTION}\\\text{AND DORSI-FLEXION}\end{array}\right)$

Fig. 38   Pronation and Supination of the Foot

61

A deformity may exist in the forefoot so that this portion of the foot is rotated about the long axis of the foot. This is referred to as pronation or supination of the forefoot. These motions take place through the tarsal joints in the mid-foot. *Pronation* exists when the first metartarsal is depressed and the lateral portion of the foot is relatively elevated. *Supination* is the term to indicate the opposite deformity and is evident by the elevation of the medial portion of the foot and depression of the lateral. These deformities are most commonly associated with bony anomalies.

Commonly the foot is abnormally deviated towards the midline in adduction with no abnormal rotary position (supination). The deformity is termed *"metatarsus adductus"* and is a congenital exaggeration of the physiologic positioning in the newborn. An abduction deformity of the forefoot without accompanying pronation is almost never seen.

When the foot is viewed from the rear the alignment of the foot is examined to determine if the *heel* is in *varus* or *valgus*. These motions take place through the talo-calcaneal (subtalar) joint.

Examination of this joint is extremely important to establish the presence of deformity and whether there is loss of motion to indicate a common source of pain. The subtalar joint is examined with the foot at right angle at the ankle to lock the talus in the mortise and diminish the amount of rocking of this bone in the ankle joint. The hindfoot is then grasped firmly in the hand and brought into the everted position and then the inverted position.

Fixed hindfoot deformities are most commonly due to underlying bony deformity or fixed soft tissue contractures while correctable malalignments are associated with muscle imbalance. Although these hindfoot deformities are seen as isolated clinical findings they are more frequently combined with mid- and forefoot anomalies.

Fig. A
ZERO STARTING
POSITION

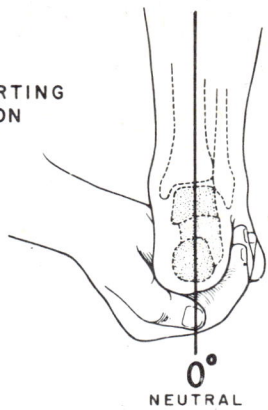

0°
NEUTRAL

Fig. B
INVERSION

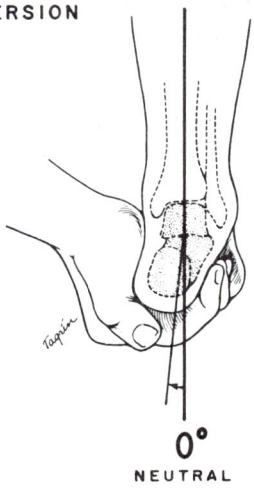

0°
NEUTRAL

Fig. C
EVERSION

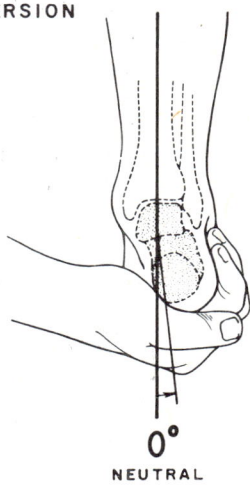

0°
NEUTRAL

Fig. 39   Motions of the Hindfoot

The classic combined deformity is the *clubfoot*. Its commonest manifestation is the foot (talipes) fixed in plantar flexion at the ankle (equinus) with the heel rolled in (varus) and the forefoot fixed in inversion; a *talipes equino-varus deformity*.

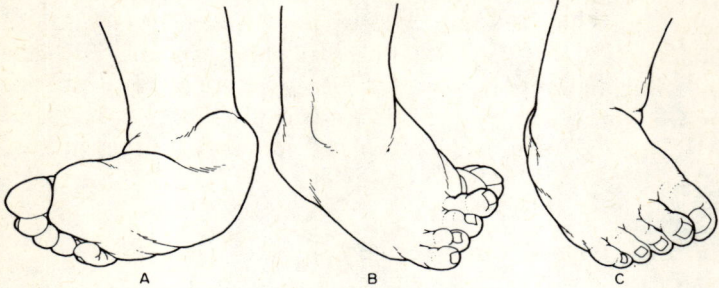

Fig. 40   Talipes Equino-varus
(A)   Plantar View   (B)   Lateral View   (C)   Dorsal View

It is more frequently a congenital deformity associated with bony malformation than acquired as a result of neurologic disease.

The reverse combined deformity with the heel dropped (calcaneus) and rolled out (valgus) and the forefoot fixed in eversion is termed *talipes calcaneo-valgus*.

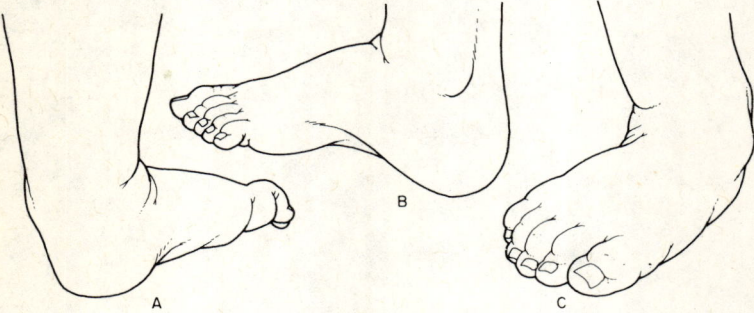

Fig. 41   Talipes Calcaneo-valgus
(A)   Posterior View   (B)   Lateral View   (C)   Dorsal View

This deformity, in contrast to the classic clubfoot, is almost always acquired and results from imbalanced muscle pull due to neurologic diseases—most commonly meningomyelocoele.

The motion of the joints of the *toes* is identified by the active and passive range of motion of the MP (metatarsalphalangeal), PIP (proximal interphalangeal), and DIP (distal inter-phalangeal) joints. The presence of any pressure points identified by the formation of calluses is recorded. Absence of toes, syndactylism, and deformities in varus or valgus should be recorded.

Fig. A 2nd. to 5th. TOES

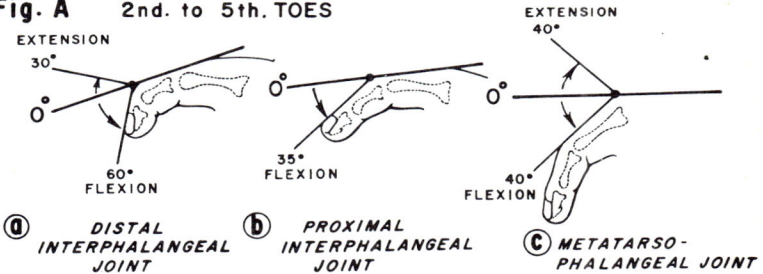

EXTENSION 30°
0°
60° FLEXION
ⓐ DISTAL INTERPHALANGEAL JOINT

0°
35° FLEXION
ⓑ PROXIMAL INTERPHALANGEAL JOINT

EXTENSION 40°
0°
40° FLEXION
ⓒ METATARSO-PHALANGEAL JOINT

0°
ABDUCTION   ABDUCTION
ADDUCTION   ADDUCTION

Fig. B

ABDUCTION and ADDUCTION

(Toe Spread)

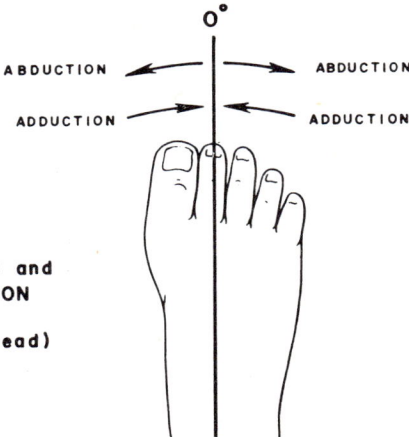

Fig. 42 Motions of the Toes

65

THE GREAT TOE

NEUTRAL
0°
FLEXION   EXTENSION
45°
70°
90°   90°

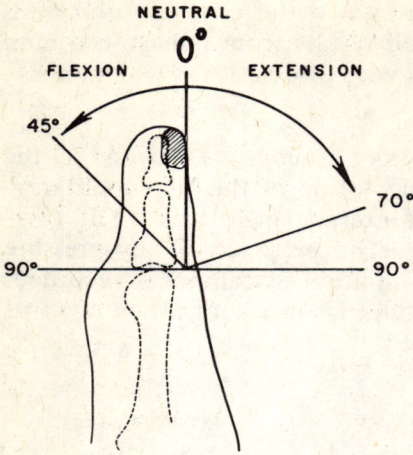

Fig. A   METATARSOPHALANGEAL JOINT

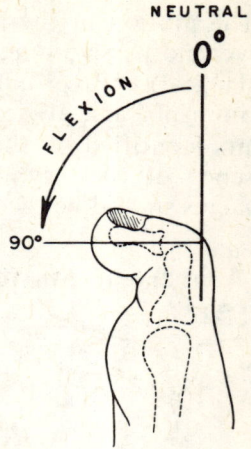

NEUTRAL
0°
FLEXION
90°

Fig. B   INTERPHALANGEAL JOINT

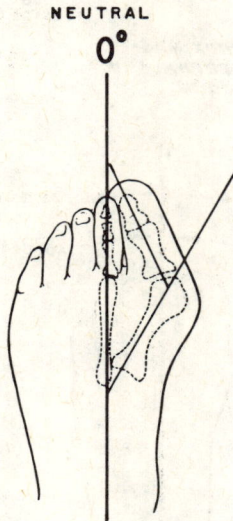

NEUTRAL
0°

Fig. C
HALLUX VALGUS

Fig. 43   Motions of the Great Toe and Hallux Valgus

Examination of the toes is done with emphasis on any deformities present. The most common deformity seen in the toes is called *hallux valgus* (bunion). The valgus refers to the deformity of the metatarsophalangeal joint of the great toe. This deformity is caused by adduction of the first metatarsal and a valgus deformity at the MP joint of the great toe. The deformity can be so severe that the great toe passes beneath the second and third toes. There is usually a bursa over the prominent medial portion of the head of the first metatarsal.

Examination of the great toe is also done to determine the degrees of motion. If motion is markedly limited and significant passive motion produces pain, it is referred to as a *hallux rigidus.*

The deformities of the other toes are usually of three types: (1) The *claw toe* deformity presents with an extension contracture of the MP joint and a flexion contracture

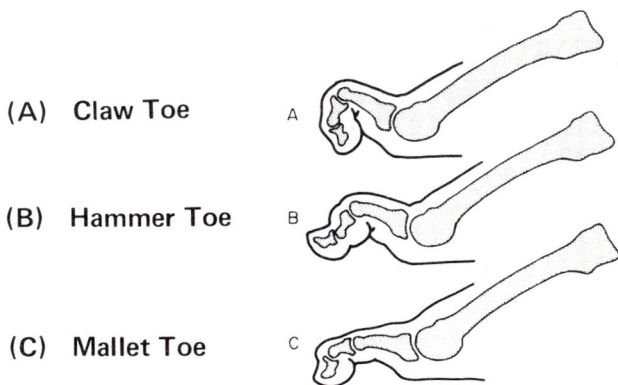

(A) Claw Toe

(B) Hammer Toe

(C) Mallet Toe

Fig. 44 Common Toe Deformities

67

of the PIP and DIP joints. Usually accompanying this deformity are callosities or corns on the dorsum of the PIP joint. If the deformity has been present for a long period, it cannot be passively corrected. The cause of this deformity is usually paralysis of the intrinsic muscles of the foot.

(2) A *hammer toe* is characteristically identified by an extension contracture of the MP joint and a flexion contracture of the PIP joint and no contracture of the DIP.

(3) The toe may have a *mallet deformity* in which the DIP joint has a flexion contracture and the other joints are relatively normal.

2. Ankle

The ankle is a modified hinge joint and the motion is that of flexion and extension at the tibio-talar joint.

The basic osseous structure is that of a mortised joint. The two malleoli, medial and lateral, fit against the body of the talus. Together with the posterior lip of the tibia they lock the talus snugly in its bed. The innate structural stability of this osseous arrangement is augmented by strong medial and lateral collateral ligaments. The medial collateral ligament passes from the medial malleolus to the navicular, calcaneus, and the talus itself. The lateral ligament consists of the anterior talofibular portion, a central slip to the calcaneus, and then a more posterior talofibular segment. These are heavy ligaments that limit inversion and eversion of the ankle. Surrounding this entire articulation is a very tough fibrous capsule.

THE ANKLE

FLEXION and EXTENSION

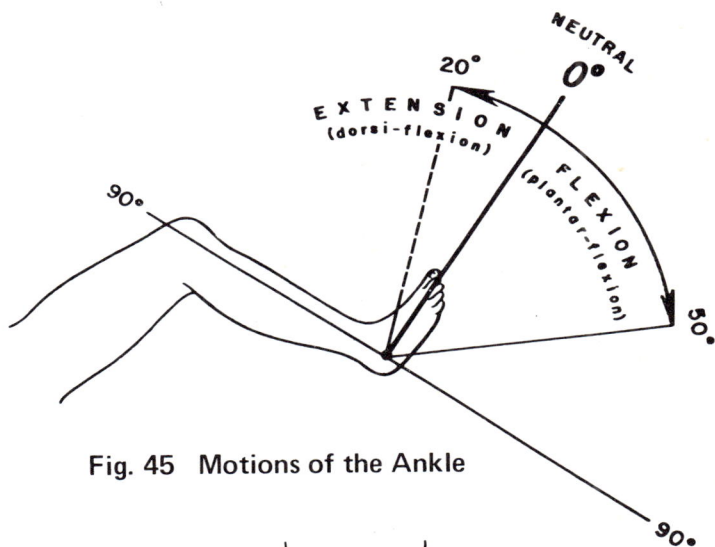

Fig. 45 Motions of the Ankle

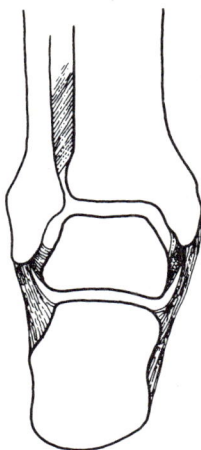

Fig. 46 Ligamentous and Osseous Stability — Ankle

69

The body of the talus has a peculiar wedge shape. It is wider in the anterior aspect of the body than it is posteriorly. Therefore, when the foot is in equinus or plantar flexed, the narrow portion of the talus is in the mortise of the ankle joint and leads to the relative instability of the ankle in this position. When the foot is dorsiflexed, the wide portion of the talus fits very snugly into the ankle joint and stabilizes the osseous structures.

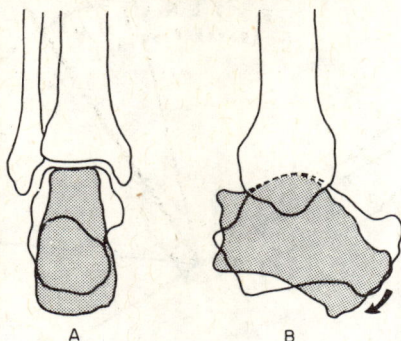

A   B

(A)   AP View—Shaded Plantar flexed   (B)   Lateral View

Fig. 47   Relative Stability of the Ankle
in Plantar—Dorsiflexion

When the ankle joint is deranged the normal motion is limited. Swelling due to joint involvement is limited by the ligaments to the region of the anterior lip of the tibia and pain is localized to this region. Swelling and tenderness distal to the malleoli indicates subtalar joint pathology—not ankle joint. The ankle is relatively infrequently involved with diseases but is one of the most common sites of injury. Rarely is the ankle aspirated diagnostically, but when indicated is most easily accomplished anteriorly with the foot in plantar flexion.

The *ankle* is the most commonly *sprained* joint in the body. The injury usually occurs with the foot in some equinus (relative tibio-talar instability) when it is subjected to a severe sudden inversion stress. The stress tears some of the fibers of the lateral collateral ligaments. The anterior segments of the ligament are more commonly damaged than the posterior. The patient immediately experiences pain and swelling in the area where the ligament has been damaged. An ecchymosis appears within two to three hours. On examination there is diffuse tenderness about the puffed lateral malleolus. There is little pain on plantar or dorsiflexion but marked pain on forced inversion.

Should the stress be severe, the lateral collateral ligament may be completely ruptured. In any "sprained" ankle it is necessary to differentiate between a true sprain and a *complete ligament tear.* Since the signs and symptoms may be quite similar, the most accurate diagnostic maneuver is an x-ray under inverting stress to identify the degree of talo-tibial instability. The ankle is anesthetized with a local anesthetic, placed in the position of equinus (if the patient describes this position at injury) and subjected to inverting stress by grasping the heel and forcefully rolling it to the limits of varus. An opening of the talus on the tibia of more than 20° is a strong indication of a ligament rupture. If there is any question about whether the opening is abnormal, a comparative stress view of the unaffected ankle should be obtained.

**Fig. 48   Stress Views
of the Ankle**

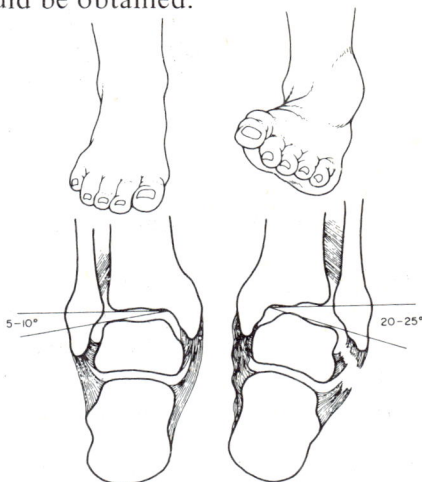

Fractures about the ankle commonly extend into and disrupt the smooth joint surfaces. If this incongruity remains after fracture healing, it will eventually lead to severe arthritic changes. Although more disabling in the weight-bearing joints, this evolution of traumatic arthritis is a potential complication of all intra-articular fractures. Particularly in sports, the ankle joint is subjected to inversion, eversion, and rotational injuries that result in fractures of the malleoli and accompanying dislocations.

The most common fracture occurring in the region of the ankle joint is the *spiral fracture* of the distal end of the fibula or the *lateral malleolus.*

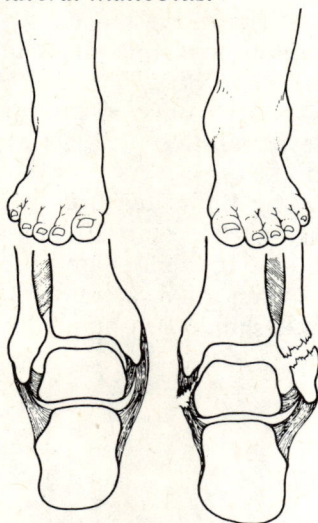

Fig. 49   Spiral Fracture—Lateral Malleolus

This is due to an eversion and external rotation of the foot. The stress may be severe enough to cause additional ligamentous injury on the medial side of the ankle. The patient presents with swelling most marked over the lateral aspect of the ankle and particularly about the lateral malleolus resembling a severe sprain. Whenever a fracture of the lateral malleolus is observed by x-ray examination, the entire length of the shaft of both bones of the leg should be examined, as the force may be transmitted up the inter-osseous membrane to the tibia. An isolated ankle x-ray may miss the diagnosis.

Fractures to both the malleoli occur with inversion and eversion injuries to the ankle joint almost always accompanied by some rotational force. The lines of fracture of the malleoli indicate whether it was an inversion or eversion injury. Should the fracture line of the medial malleolus be transverse and the lateral malleolus oblique, it indicates an eversion external rotational force while a transverse line through the lateral malleolus and the reverse points to an inversion and internal rotational force. With disruption of the bony mortise caused by these *bimalleolar fractures* there are varying degrees of lateral displacement (subluxation) of the talus in the mortise.

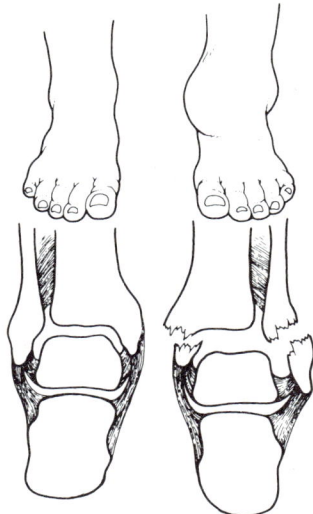

Fig. 50   Bimalleolar Fracture—Subluxation—Ankle

On examination there is generalized swelling, all motion is painful, ecchymosis is seen early, and the entire ankle is thickened or spread.

73

Finally, if the injury is sufficiently forceful, additional plantar flexion of the foot may result in a fracture through the posterior lip of the tibia (called the third malleolus) resulting in three distinct fracture lines—one through the lateral malleolus; one through the medial malleolus; and one through the posterior lip of the tibia. The talus usually dislocates posteriorly with this *trimalleolar fracture*.

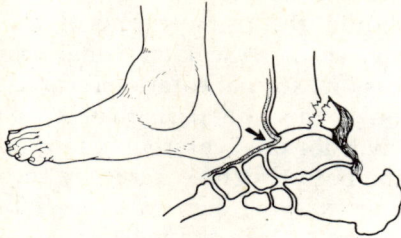

Fig. 51   Trimalleolar Fracture—Dislocation—Ankle

On examination this ankle is markedly swollen, ecchymotic, and fixed in the deformed position. The foot may be set to the side and the distal end of the tibia bulges forward due to dislocation. The anterior displacement may occlude the dorsalis pedis and the foot may be white and pulseless. With this deformity, if there will be any appreciable delay in x-ray, gentle attempts at reduction should be done to reduce the dislocation and restore the blood supply.

3. Leg

The leg is that portion of the lower extremity between the knee and the ankle. On inspection particular attention should be paid to the contours of the calf. When this muscle group is thin, it represents atrophy. While a symmetrical atrophy is easily recognizable, bilateral atrophy (presenting as spindly calves or *"stork legs"*) may be less obvious. Calf atrophy may be due to disuse or paralysis. Hypertrophy of the calves, particularly in relation to the thighs, is a

74

physical sign suggestive of muscular dystrophy. Unilateral hypertrophy of the calf is extremely uncommon and unequal calf size usually suggests the smaller is atrophic.

Viewed from the front the leg may reveal a medial or lateral angular deformity while viewing it from the side determines whether there is an anterior bow. This gentle curve and the sharp anterior crest of the tibia may suggest *"sabre shins."*

Children are normally *"pigeon-toed."* This position is contributed to by three components; 1. metatarsus adductus of the foot, 2. internal tibial torsion of the leg, and 3. anteversion of the hip (next section). The degree of torsion is estimated by placing the knee in 90° of flexion and holding the patella forward. An imaginary line between the medial and lateral malleoli should strike an angle of 30° relative to the transverse axis of the knee. This is estimated by sighting down the tibia while palpating the malleoli.

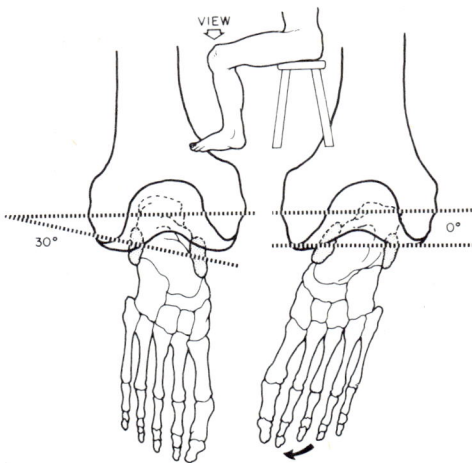

Fig. 52 Estimating Tibial Torsion

"Tibial torsion" is used to clinically describe an excessive internal torsional rotation of the tibia. This physiologic deformity in young children commonly spontaneously

corrects by age six as do the other components of "toe-ing-in". Progressive or unresponsive tibial torsion may mean a pathologic softening and deforming of the tibia under normal physiologic stress.

The leg is measured in length from the joint line to the medial malleolus and is measured in girth by defining the largest circumference of the calf. This is variable and at times requires two to three measurements in different areas.

The observation of the leg should be concerned with identifying the presence of swelling, most commonly seen in the lower third. One should also be aware of the distribution of the hair on the leg, its absence indicating chronic circulatory disturbance. Scars over the anterior crest of the tibia are troublesome and should be recorded if present. The leg is prone to ulcer formation and the presence of these and discoloration should be noted.

Palpation of the leg should take advantage of the subcutaneous position of the tibia. This bone can be palpated from the knee joint down to the ankle. Any deformities, tenderness, or angulation of this bone can be readily identified by palpation. Palpation of the leg also should include testing the consistency of the triceps surae; any increment in firmness or rubbery consistency may suggest muscular dystrophy.

Open fractures are seen frequently in the tibia because this bone is just subcutaneous and minimal deformation or laceration perforates the skin overlying the bone. The wound may vary from a small laceration oozing dark blood to a huge avulsion with several inches of bone exposed. In any open fracture, regardless of the extent of the soft tissue wound, an important consideration is the prevention of subsequent infection and osteomyelitis. Thus small lacerations over any fracture must be carefully examined to see if the wound communicates with the fracture site. Helpful tip-offs are (1) Fat globules from the marrow admixed with the oozing blood, (2) Palpable bone (remember wear gloves! and masks!!) just beneath the adjacent skin, and

(3) Presence of air in the fracture site on x-ray. If communication is still uncertain, probe gently with a STERILE instrument. If still in doubt treat as an open fracture.

Since all open fractures require immediate debridement in the operating room environment, rapid assessment of the pulses, sensation, and motor function in the leg and foot should be done accurately and recorded so as to not delay treatment, which will in time, increase the incidence of osteomyelitis.

The term *"shin splints"* at present defies a universally accepted definition except pain somewhere between the knee and ankle following exertion. Pain in the muscle mass in the proximal anterior lateral aspect of the leg following long running or walking is considered by some to be shin splints. This complaint is due to a transient ischemia of the anterior leg muscle group and is usually relieved by rest. Extreme exertion beyond the point of pain or acute occlusive vascular problems may cause severe intra-compartmental ischemia and edema of these muscles causing *"anterior compartment syndrome."* Clinically this syndrome is manifest by a woody firm resistance to palpation and later by hypesthesia between the first and second toes. Plantar flexion of the foot and toes causes severe pain. Intra-compartmental pressure measurement of 80 mm of water or more indicates the need for immediate surgical decompression. Individuals participating in running may complain of pain posteromedial to the distal third of the tibia accompanied by mild swelling and pain on dorsiflexion and eversion of the foot and hyperextension of the great toe. This is another form of "shin splints" caused by tendinitis of the tibialis posterior, flexor hallucis longus and common flexor digitorium. This condition must be differentiated from a stress fracture of the tibia or fibula.

4. The Knee

The knee is described as a hinge joint. Although the tibia does extend and flex on the condyles of the femur, resembling the motion of a hinge, the tibia actually glides anteriorly and posteriorly about the eccentric condyles of the femur around a shifting center of motion. The final few degrees of full extension is accompanied by 15° of internal rotation of the femur on the tibia when the foot is planted on the ground. In the actual examination of the knee, with the patient supine and the femur fixed, the last 15° of extension is conversely accompanied by an external rotation of the tibia on the fixed femur; this is called the screw-home mechanism. The knee joint is actively extended by the large quadriceps muscle which takes up the anterior, medial, and lateral aspects of the thigh; the quadriceps inserts into the patella and through this bone and the patellar tendon into the tibial tubercle of the leg. This insertion is strongly enhanced by fibrous medial and lateral retinacula which are "tendinous" extensions of the vastus medialis and vastus lateralis bellies of the quadriceps. This complex, that is, the quadriceps, patella, and the patellar tendon, and medial and lateral retinacula, composes what is termed the extensor mechanism. This strong extensor mechanism greatly stabilizes the knee when the quadriceps is fully contracted. The major function of the quadriceps and extensor mechanism is to act as a decelerator, not an extensor. As one runs, or walks down stairs, the extensor mechanism, (the quadriceps) contracts, pushing the patella in a posterior direction against the femur, decelerating the anterior motion of the body weight, and preventing one from falling forward. Weakness or momentary spinal reflex relaxation of the quadriceps causes the knee to give way and allows one to fall because of the loss of this deceleration. So, this strong extensor mechanism greatly stabilizes the knee when the quadriceps is fully contracted. The knee is flexed by the hamstrings and the gastrocnemius. However, they also control the rotation of the tibiofemoral joint by their

78

insertion into the sides of the tibia and they greatly enhance the stability of the knee joint when the knee is weight bearing in flexion by their insertions into the posteromedial and posterolateral capsular ligaments of the knee.

The stability of the knee is enhanced by the contour of the two condyles of the femur fitting into the depressions in the plateau of the tibia, the firm apposition of these two bony structures by the pull of the large anterior and posterior muscle groups, and finally by the heavy ligaments and joint capsule surrounding this joint. The menisci act as wedges around the periphery of the tibial surfaces, that prevent the round femoral condyles from slipping off the top of the tibia. The ligaments act as hinges and provide *static stability*. The muscles crossing the knee joint provide dynamic *stability*.

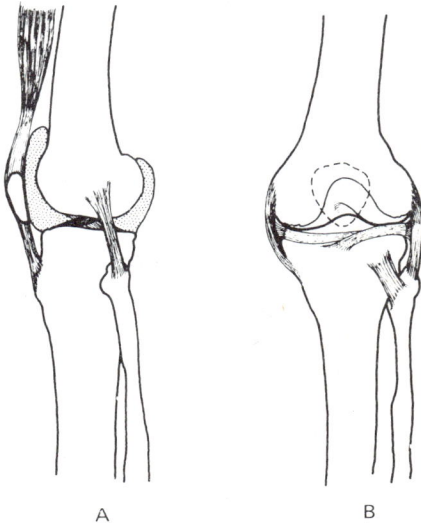

A   B

Fig. 53

(A) Lateral view—
Major Ligaments,
Muscles, and Capsule

(B) Frontal view—
Major Ligaments
and Menisci

79

HYPEREXTENSION

0°
NEUTRAL

FLEXION

135°

90°

0° NEUTRAL

30°

135°   90°

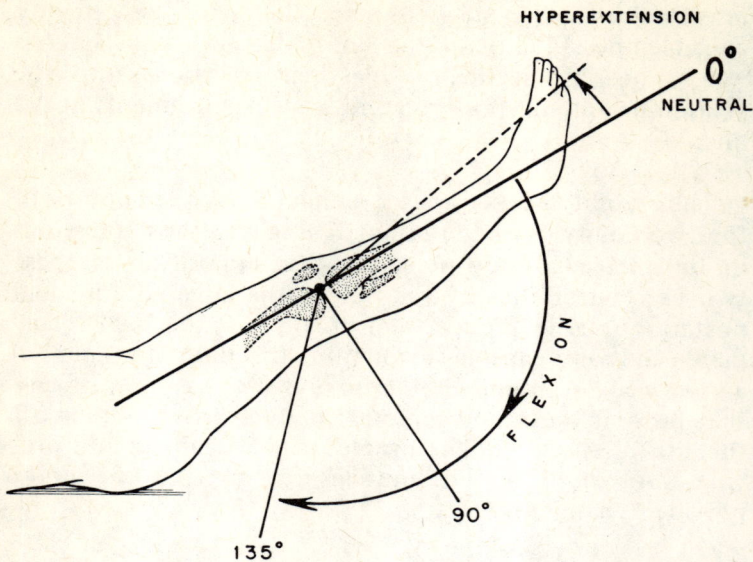

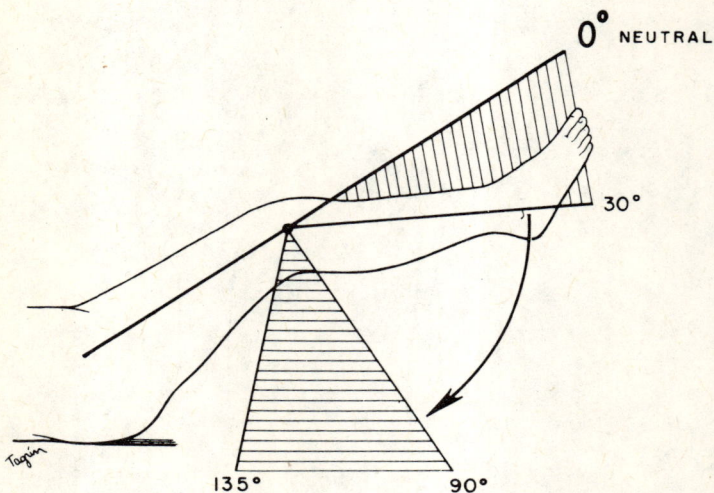

Fig. 53 (C) Ranges of Knee Motion

The knee has the largest joint cavity in the body. This cavity starts two inches above the patella forming a reflected synovial sac called the *suprapatellar pouch*. This communicates with the articulation between the femur, tibia, and patella which has medial and lateral reflections of synovial tissue starting at the osteochondral junctions of all bones involved. This synovium sometimes has a concentric fold just proximal to the patella called the *suprapatellar plica*. The joint cavity also extends posteriorly to cover the condyles of the femur and the tibia.

Knee joint motion is recorded as $0°$ for complete extension, and flexion is measured from this point. Hyperextension is recorded as minus degrees.

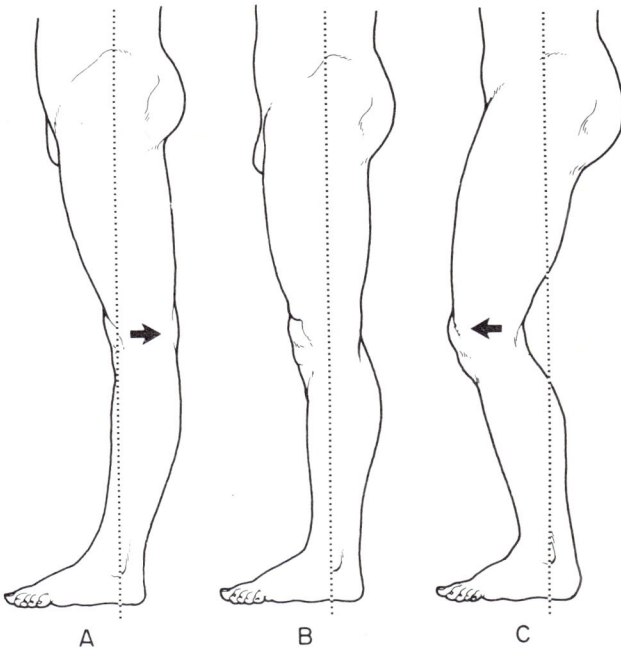

Fig. 54 (A) Recurvatum Deformity (B) Normal (C) Flexion Contracture

Knee examination commences with the patient standing and one views the knee from the front, that is, in the anteroposterior plane. Alignment is normal when the leg is straight with a mild valgus; bowleg or tibia vara when present is usually most prominent in the proximal tibia; knock-knee or genu valgum occurs at the level of the knee joint itself. Then viewing the knee from the side we inspect for incomplete extension (flexion contracture) or *recurvatum* deformity (back-knee).

From the rear, the popliteal adiposities (popliteal fat pads) are examined to see if they are equal, or if one side is larger indicating possibly a *popliteal (Baker's) cyst*. During this inspection both knees are evaluated for any comparative abnormality of contour, that is, abnormal masses or swelling.

The patella is a common (but frequently overlooked) source of knee symptoms. To examine the patella, the patient is asked to sit on the examining table with the legs

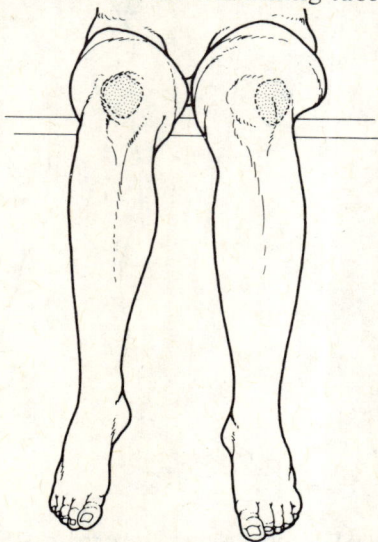

Fig. 55 Normal and laterally displaced patellae

hanging loosely off the table in about 80 to 90° of flexion with the knees held close together. Viewed from the front, the patellae should face forward rather than somewhat off to the side.

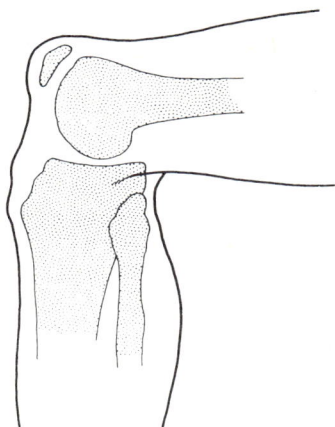

Fig. 56   Patella Alta

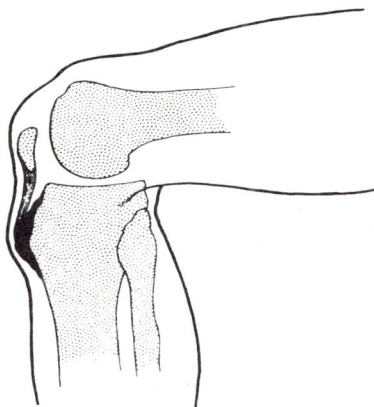

Fig. 57   Prominent Tibial Tubercle (Osgood-Schlatter's)

Observed from the side, the patallae should lie squarely on the end of the femur rather than facing somewhat toward the ceiling. When the patella is situated obliquely with the knee flexed, the position is called *patella alta* — a high riding patella. This position is frequently associated with a concavity in the soft tissue just proximal to the upper pole of the patella. Patellae pointing laterally (seen from the front) and facing more toward the ceiling (seen from the side), have a concavity proximal to the upper pole which indicates that lateral subluxation is a strong possibility.

While viewing the knees from the side, the tibial tubercles may be compared for prominence and evidence of unusual callosities. Enlargement, particularly in adolescents, may indicate *Osgood-Schlatters disease*.

While the patient is sitting, the thighs are checked for atrophy or loss of tone. The patient is asked to extend the leg to 45° of flexion. A concavity medial to the upper part

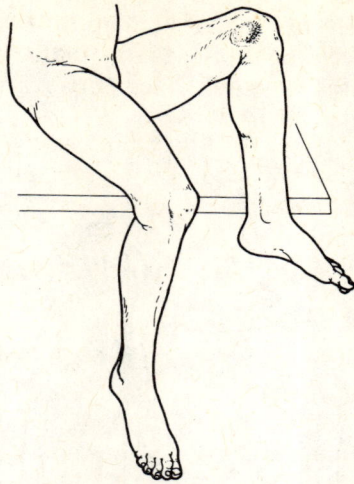

Fig. 58   Atrophic Vastus Medialis

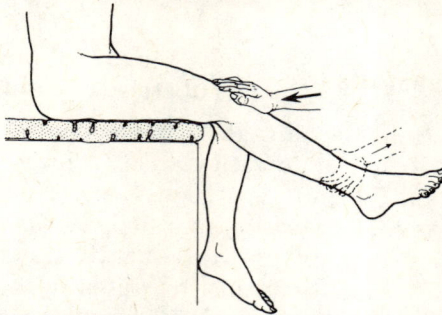

Fig. 59   Examining for Subpatellar Crepitation

of the patella and a prominent edge or outline of the quadriceps tendon indicate significant atrophy or congential dysplasia of the distal end of the vastus medialis. Congenital dysplasia of this muscle is frequent in patellar subluxation.

The patient now extends the legs completely to 0° and then flexes them to a right angle. The motion is watched to see if the rhythm is normal and the patella moves smoothly. This active range of motion is repeated while the examiner pushes the patella firmly against the underlying femoral condyles. Pain and grating indicate irregularities (degeneration) in the articular cartilage of the patella *(chondromalacia)*.

While the patient is still sitting, the examiner supports the patient's leg (flexed 30°) to relax the quadriceps and further checks patellar stability by attempting to push the patella laterally. An abnormal amount of lateral displacement, pain, and apprehension indicate a *subluxing patella*.

Injuries to the knee (particularly in athletics) as well as arthritic changes are manifested by swelling, limited motion, instability, and *"catching"* or *"locking."* These findings may conveniently be sought with the patient in the supine position.

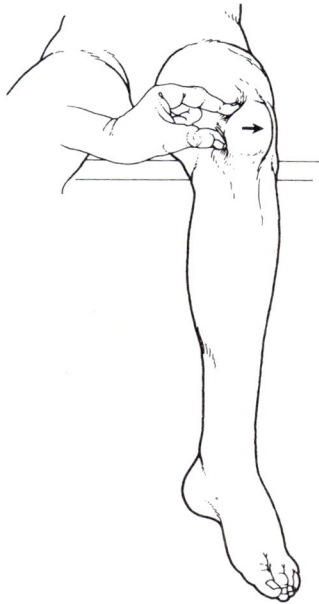

Fig. 60   Examining for Patellar Stability

With the patient lying supine, note whether both knees come completely straight or if one lacks some extension. A mild limitation of extension may now be noticeable when it was not evident previously. Gingerly force a limited knee into complete extension and determine whether this maneuver is painful. Traumatic or degenerative tears of the menisci or other internal derangement may prevent complete extension. Such *"locking"* is usually accompanied by quadriceps weakness *("giving way")*.

Again observe the thighs for comparative size and contour. Muscle atrophy or loss of tone will cause one to appear flat, the normal to appear rounded. Measure the circumference of each thigh with a tape measure at an equal distance from a fixed bony landmark, such as, the top of the lateral tibial plateau (as illustrated). The patella (more commonly used) is not as good a base line as its position is more variable. Seven inches is a good proximal point to measure possible thigh atrophy as this is usually above the suprapatellar pouch and thus above the point of possible knee joint distension. The circumference of the knee and the calf may be measured in a like manner.

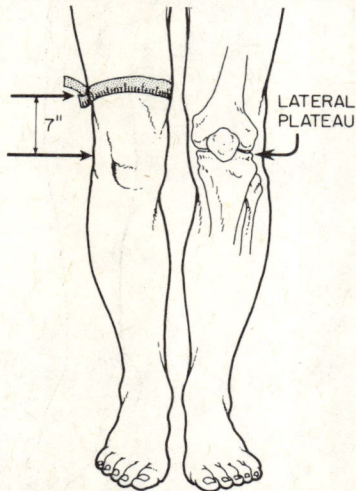

Fig. 61 Measuring Thigh Atrophy

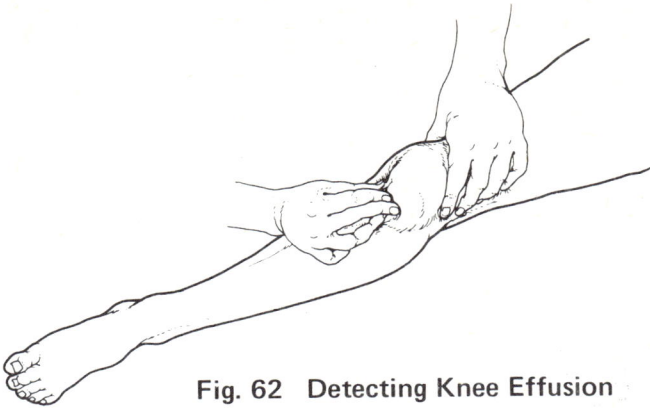

Fig. 62 Detecting Knee Effusion

If the knee is swollen, an effort should be made to distinguish whether the excess fluid is in the joint (deep to the patella) or in the large bursa that lies superficial to the patella. This distinction is sought by applying moderate pressure with one hand over the suprapatellar pouch (forcing any intraarticular fluid into the joint) and simultaneously pressing the patella toward the underlying femoral condyle. *Ballotment* of the patella will occur if the swelling is within the joint. If the prepatellar pouch is swollen, this sack of fluid can usually be outlined with the palpating fingers demonstrating the patellar edges beneath it. An additional clue is that intraarticular swelling is more likely to be accompanied by more limitation of extension than is usual with prepatellar bursitis *(housemaid's knee)*.

While examining for an effusion, the suprapatellar pouch is felt carefully for hard, movable loose bodies that usually feel like an olive pit.

The patella may be further examined using the palm of the hand to force the patella against the femoral condyles while rocking the patella to and fro in both the longitudinal and transverse planes. Grating and pain indicate chondromalacia of the patella.

87

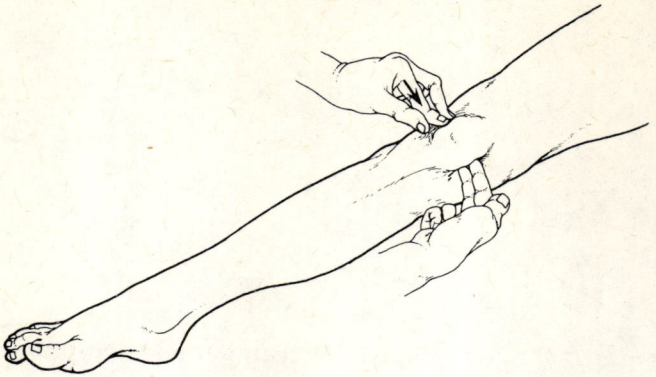

Fig. 63   Examining for Subpatellar Discomfort

The most common area of *chondromalacia* (pain) is beneath the medial facet of the patella and is specifically sought by displacing the patella medially and pressing the forefinger firmly against the articular face of the medial facet.

Acute tenderness over the capsule medial and distal to the patella indicates a strain of this fibrous tissue, most commonly occurring when the patella has subluxed. Very localized tenderness over the medial femoral epicondyle indicates a sprain of the tibial collateral ligament at this attachment.

The patient is now requested to contract the quadriceps bilaterally. A goniometer is centered over the patella with one arm lying over the patellar tendon and the other arm pointing toward the anterior superior iliac spine. The normal angulation is usually 10° of lateral deviation. Angulation of 15° to 20° is considered abnormal and is called the "Q" *angle*. Any increase calls attention to a potential lateral subluxation of the patella. Confirmatory signs are the illusion of a double patella due to an unusually

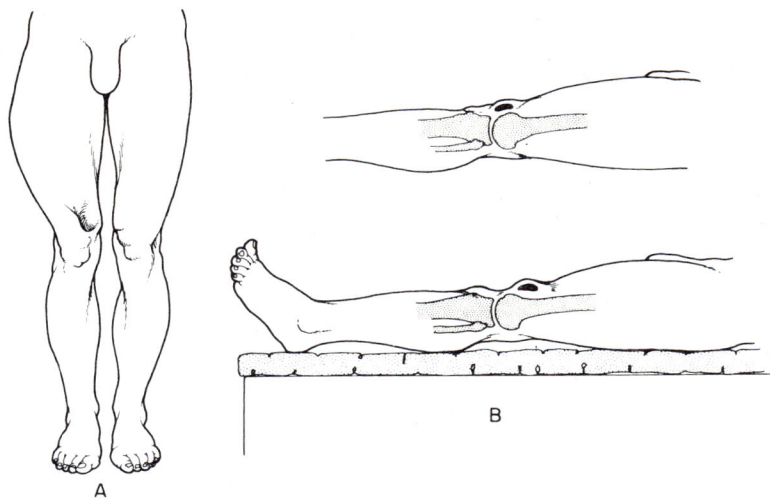

Fig. 64 (A) Hypertrophic Vastus Lateralis
(B) Normal and "Camelback" Patellar Contours

prominent infrapatellar fat pad (the *"camelback" sign*) and hypertrophy of the vastus lateralis which pulls the patella into the subluxed position on extension.

The presence of internal derangement and ligamentous instability of the knee is best checked while the patient is supine. The knee is flexed to 90°, the hip flexed 45°, and the foot planted on the examining table. Before these evaluations, several observations are conveniently made with the knee in this position. Puffiness, or even a large mass, at the lateral joint line of the involved knee compared to the normal is indicative of a possible tear of the lateral meniscus. A slightly edematous feel and pain here give more support to the possibility of a torn lateral meniscus.

In this position, the normal small concavities on either side of the patellar tendon are evident, and minimal

89

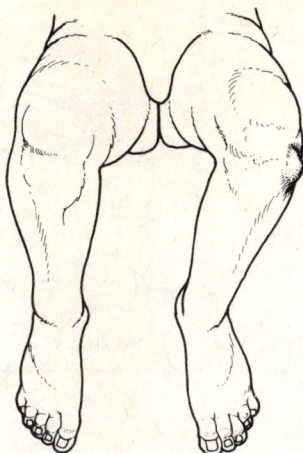

Fig. 65   Distended Lateral Joint Line (from above)

amount of swelling not previously evident may be demonstrated by loss of these concavities.

Palpate both the medial joint line over the medial meniscus and the region of the *pes anserinus* just distal to the joint line for tenderness. Any swelling distal to the joint and tenderness to palpation indicate inflammation of the underlying bursa which can mimic all the symptoms and disability of a torn meniscus of the knee.

Fingertip palpation over the specific anatomical structures of the knee is very helpful in the localization of pathology.

Internal derangement of the knee (loose bodies and loose flaps of meniscal cartilage) is sought for by *McMurray's test.* The knee is moved into full flexion and full extension with the tibia held in internal rotation for one cycle and external rotation for another and both are repeated. Limitation of acute flexion with pain may indicate a torn meniscus posteriorly. A positive sign is a "popping" in or about the knee joint. Such popping,

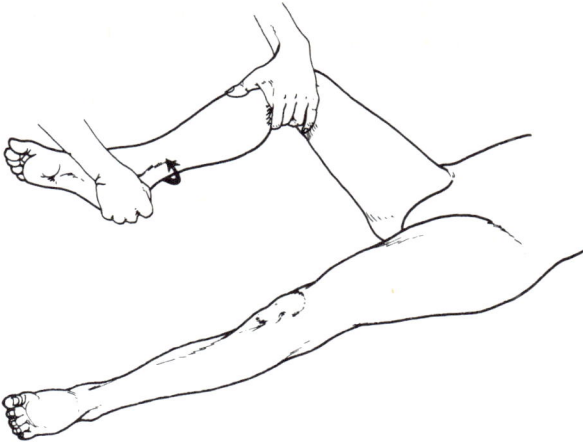

Fig. 66 McMurray's Test

however, may be normal when caused by a tendon passing over a bony prominence. Popping is indicative of a meniscus tear when the meniscus can be felt to "lurch" simultaneously beneath the palpating finger of the examiner.

Genu varum and/or *internal tibial torsion,* if previously detected, needs a little more scrutiny while the patient is still supine. This is particularly true of the very young and the elderly. Tibial torsion is often associated with genu varum. With pure varus deformity the ankles cross with the feet pointing up when the medial femoral condyles are touching, whereas coexisting tibial torsion produces relatively less crossing of the ankles with the feet tending to point across the midline. It is quite important in a patient whose knee is to be surgically realigned to be aware of how much of the deformity is bending (varus) and how much is twisting (torsional).

Each hip is now passively moved through a full range of motion. It is embarrassing to "examine" the painful knee of a high school athlete, obtain normal knee x-rays repeatedly and even to inject the knee just hoping for therapeutic relief, and then have one of your orthopaedic

91

colleagues examine the boy and find a slipped capital femoral epiphysis. Hip pathology frequently is manifested at first as referred knee pain. This is particularly true in children when the complaints are medial (obturator nerve). In the elderly, a swollen knee may be on the basis of chronic strain secondary to hip pathology. This in no way implies a routine radiographic study of the hips is indicated in the evaluation of knee disability. It does indicate that hip evaluation is a routine part of the regional knee examination.

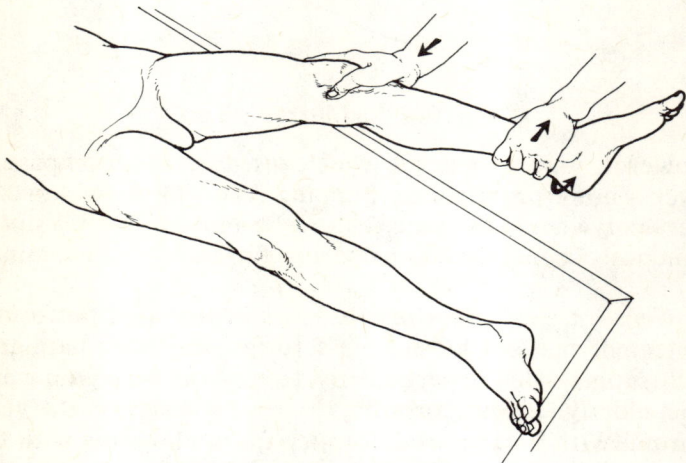

Fig. 67   Abduction Stress Test

The *abduction stress test* for a tear of the ligaments of medial compartment is performed by sightly abducting the hip, moving the thigh toward the side of the table, bending the knee off the side to about 30°, pressing against the outside of the knee with one hand while grasping the inside of the distal leg with the other, and abducting gently only to the point of pain. The examiner needs to walk around to the other side of the table and examine the supposedly normal knee in a like manner. In fact, it is far better to examine the normal knee first so the patient may know what to expect and thus be less apprehensive when the injured knee is examined. Demonstrated instability of all ligaments should be graded one, two, or three plus (mild, moderate, and severe respectively), or the deformity produced should be measured in degrees. Each examiner's mild or moderate will not be exactly the same, but as one becomes experienced, they will be close enough for meaningful communication if the testing techniques have been the same. Furthermore, it is not the objective of examination to force ligamentous instability to its maximum, as it is often quite painful. It is only important to determine the degree of instability in order to make a decision relative to the desirable treatment.

Abduction stress is next applied in a similar manner but with the knee in 0° extension, or in whatever degree of recurvatum the opposite normal knee may demonstrate. A medial opening or "give" of a moderate or 2+ rating at 0° extension indicates an associated tear of the posterior cruciate ligament in the acute injury.

The anterior and posterior *drawer tests* are performed with the patient supine, the hip flexed 45°, the knee flexed about 90°, the foot planted on the examining table, and the examiner's buttock sitting partially on the forefoot. The upper leg is grasped with both hands with the forefingers against the hamstrings to note any contraction and resultant resistance to an effective testing. Now, a gentle to and fro push and pull is exerted on the distally fixed leg. This examination is carried out with the tibia first externally rotated, then in neutral rotation, then internally rotated, with the rotation controlled by sitting on the foot.

In a positive anterior drawer test there is a forward jog or movement with comparative abnormal prominence of the upper tibia anteriorly. In a positive posterior drawer test there is an abnormal backward displacement of the upper tibia with an anterior prominence of the distal

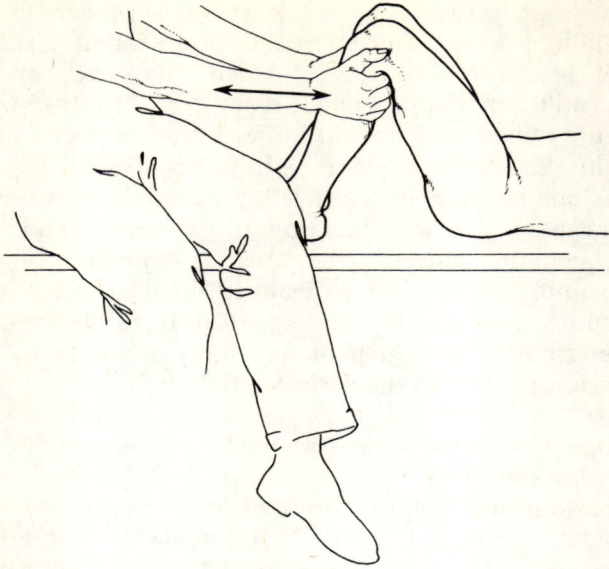

Fig. 68   Drawer Test

femur and patella. Classically described as a test for anterior and posterior cruciate integrity, there are other ligaments and fascial bands which are responsible for knee stability in this anteroposterior plane. The part these structures play is dependent upon the rotational position of the tibia on the femur during the drawer maneuver.

If the posterior cruciate ligament is intact and the positive anterior drawer sign can be demonstrated with the tibia externally rotated, the displacement is in reality an anteromedial rotational instability. With the tibia in neutral rotation, if the anterior drawer test is positive, both tibial condyles may appear to come forward equally, or the lateral tibial condyle may appear to come forward a bit more than the medial. This positive anterior drawer test with the tibia in neutral rotation indicates that there is probably an anterolateral rotatory instability.   Con-

94

versely with the tibia internally rotated, the anterior drawer test will be normal as long as the posterior cruciate ligament is intact, regardless of how many or how severely other ligaments are torn. In addition, the anterior drawer test can be positive without a tear of the anterior cruciate ligament. When the tibia is externally rotated, the medial ligaments as well as the anterior cruciate play a part in stabilizing the knee. In this position, insufficient medial ligaments alone (positive abduction stress sign) will permit the medial tibial plateau to shift forward. The degree of severity of this anteromedial rotational instability is increased by an associated tear of the anterior cruciate ligament. Many investigators believe that the anterior drawer test will be positive only when the anterior cruciate ligament is torn.

Patients with this disability commonly complain of *"giving way"* or having the knee buckle when weight is borne on it. This giving way, associated with many knee problems, is usually due to weakness of the quadriceps (extension) mechanism and its inability to support body weight. The weakness in turn is the result of atrophy of the muscle due to disuse.

There is, however, a peculiar type of giving way that may be associated with anterior cruciate insufficiency. This giving way is precipitated by sudden directional change while walking or running and is the result of forward subluxation of the lateral plateau of the tibia on the femur. Described by McIntosh and Galway, this is known, because of its frequency while playing sports, as the "pivot-shift" sign. It is the opposite of the anteromedial rotational instability in that the subluxation occurs as the knee goes into extension with the tibia internally rotated. When the knee is subsequently flexed, the subluxation reduces with an audible "clunk" at about 30°. The subluxation presents on physical examination as a positive anterior drawer sign with the tibia in neutral rotation. The internal rotational component of this instability may be demonstrated by alternately flexing and extending the knee while simultaneously holding the tibia internally rotated at the ankle with one hand and applying a valgus stress on the knee and a forward thrust on the proximal tibia with the other hand. At about 30° there is a visible and audible "clunk" that reproduces the patient's symptoms. The maneuvers of flexing and extending the knee while internally and externally rotating the tibia are closely similar to those maneuvers of the McMurray test and in anterolateral rotatory instability when the patient and the examiner feels the "clunk", the patient may complain of simultaneous medial joint pain thereby raising the distinct possibility of confusing anterolateral rotatory instability with popping and slipping of a torn medial meniscus.

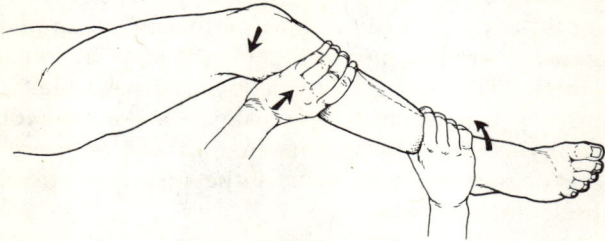

Fig. 69   Extending, Internally Rotating, and Lifting the Tibia Forward

The other lateral ligament instabilities are difficult to evaluate. The adduction stress test is performed in a manner exactly the opposite of the abduction test. When it is positive it is indicative of a tear of the lateral ligaments of the knee. The normal or physiological looseness of the lateral compartment causes acute tears to be missed clinically. In the presence of a history of the knee being forced into varus and tenderness over the lateral ligaments, the lateral stabilities of the patient's injured and normal knee must be carefully compared. There are two additional helpful diagnostic tests which indicate tears of the arcuate ligament complex in the posterolateral corner of the knee. The external rotational

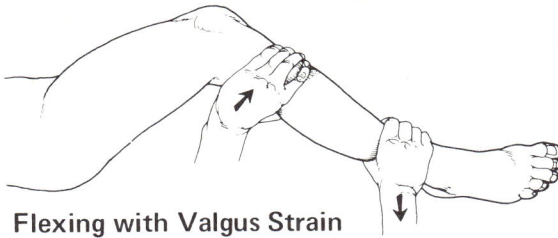

Fig. 70 Flexing with Valgus Strain
Produces the "Pivot-Shift" clunk

recurvatum test is performed with the patient supine
and the examiner standing at the foot of the examining
table and lifting the lower limb by the toes or by cupping
the heel or ankle in the palm of the hand so as to avoid
controlling rotation. As extension of the knee occurs
keep a sharp eye on the proximal tibia to observe any
excess of external rotation and recurvatum. Perform the
test on the opposite normal knee for comparison. A positive external rotational recurvatum test is often as subtle
as the patient's symptoms. It is positive when the proximal
tibia goes into comparably greater recurvatum and simultaneously externally rotates beyond the point of the
screw-home mechanism, thereby giving a feeling of no end-
point or absence of stable locking in extension. Tibia
vara is also evident.

The posterolateral drawer test is positive when the
posterior push on the tibia in mild external rotation produces an excessive posterior displacement and a further
external rotation of the proximal tibia, suggesting a
posterior subluxation of the entire proximal tibia. The
examiner immediately suspects a posterior cruciate ligament laxity until he more closely inspects the action of
the proximal tibia and notices that the external rotation
is associated with more subluxation of the lateral tibial
plateau than of the medial tibial plateau. For further
differentiation, the degree of posterior subluxation is
tested with the tibia internally rotated. In the case of
posterior cruciate ligament laxity, the tibia remains displaced posteriorly — a finding not present if the posterior
cruciate is intact.

97

5. Hip and Thigh

The hip joint is one of the most stable joints of the body. It is a ball and socket joint which has innate stability due to the osseous structures. The head of the femur fits into the acetabulum and is held snuggly by the capsule. Stability of the hip joint is also greatly aided by the vacuum effect of a ball and socket joint resisting distraction. Finally, stability is aided by the balance of adjacent muscles about the joint.

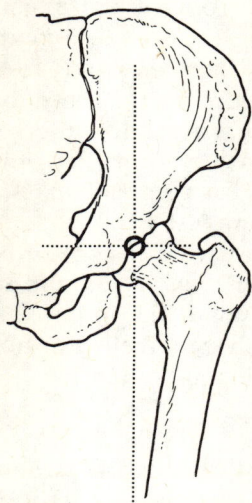

Fig. 71

Frontal View—Hip Joint   **Fig. 72   The Hip Flexors**

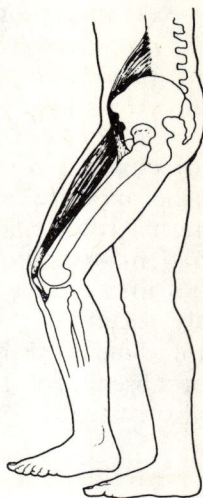

Figure 71 shows the relationship of the head of the femur to the acetabulum—the axis of motion is through the center of the head of the femur. The laterally directed femoral neck displaces the entire shaft of the femur lateral to this axis, an important consideration when discussing the function of the muscles of the region.

The hip joint is controlled by the large bulky surrounding muscles. These are divided into anatomic groups. The anterior muscles flex the thigh at the hip and the most important muscle in this group is the iliopsoas.

98

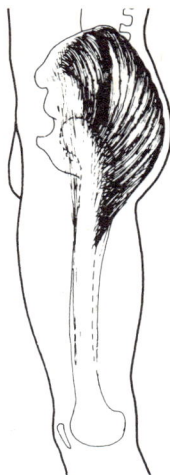

Fig. 73 Hip Extensor   Fig. 74 Hip Abductor

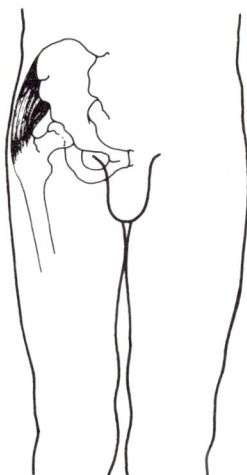

The rectus femoris of the quadriceps assists this muscle in hip flexion. Of lesser importance are the tensor fascia lata and sartorius.

The posterior hip muscles are comprised principally of the gluteal muscles. The gluteus maximus extends the thigh at the hip.

Lateral to the gluteus maximus is the gluteus medius muscle, the principal hip abductor.

Besides abducting the thigh, the gluteus medius stabilizes the pelvis in the stance phase of gait, the anatomic origin becoming the functional insertion and the insertion becoming the functional origin.

On the medial side of the thigh extending to the pelvis is another large mass of muscles called the adductors. These muscles arise from the inferior pubic and ischial rami and insert into the posterior medial aspect of the femur throughout most of its length.

As noted earlier in the general examination, considerable information about deformity, muscle function, and

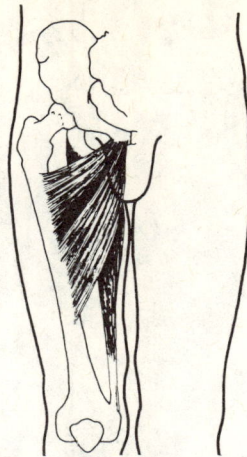

Fig. 75　Hip Adductors

pain about the hip can be obtained by observing the patient's gait. Examination of the hip begins by observing
for atrophy of the thigh. Atrophy of the proximal thigh
suggests chronic hip disease. This is measured circumferentially as far proximal as possible. Atrophy of the gluteal
muscles presents as flattening of the buttock and loss of
muscle tone on palpation.

Examination of the bony landmarks about the hip
assists in determining the presence of deformity.

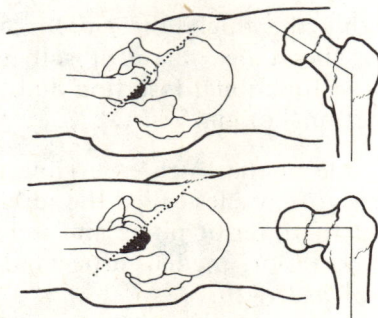

Fig. 76　Nelaton's Line

Nelaton's Line: Nelaton's line is a line drawn between the ischial tuberosity and the anterior superior iliac spine. As indicated by the dotted line in Figure 76, palpating the trochanter well above Nelaton's line indicates either a dislocation of the hip or *coxa vara.* Coxa vara is a deformity in which the femoral neck droops over medially thus decreasing the angle between the neck and shaft.

Palpation of the region of the hip seeks to determine the anatomic location of tenderness. The most common area of tenderness related to the hip joint is in the groin with pain radiating down the medial thigh. Tenderness over the greater trochanter suggests superficial trochanteric bursitis. Tenderness deep in the buttock may have several causes—sciatic nerve irritation, hip joint distention, deep gluteal bursitis, etc.

Attention is now directed to the range of motion of the hip joint. This examination is done on a firm examining table. The opposite thigh is flexed on the abdomen to eliminate the lumbar lordosis and to insure that only hip flexion is being determined and not motion at the lumbosacral joint.

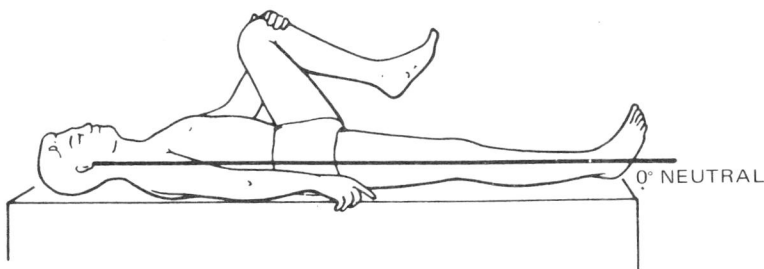

Fig. 77   Locking the Pelvis and Lumbar Spine prior to Estimating Hip Flexion

The opposite thigh is held in the flexed position by the patient or the examiner. The hip under observation is now allowed to extend to the neutral position. Failure to reach this position indicates a hip flexion contracture.

101

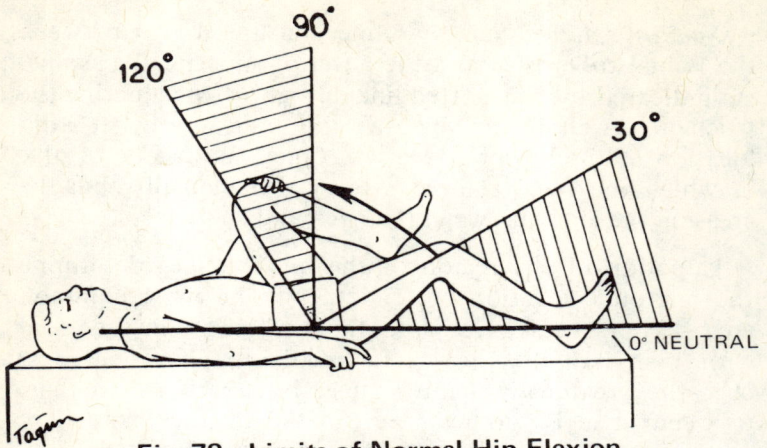

Fig. 78 Limits of Normal Hip Flexion

The range of hip flexion is demonstrated by flexing the hip being observed. The limit of flexion is determined by movement of the pelvis indicated by motion of the contralateral hip.

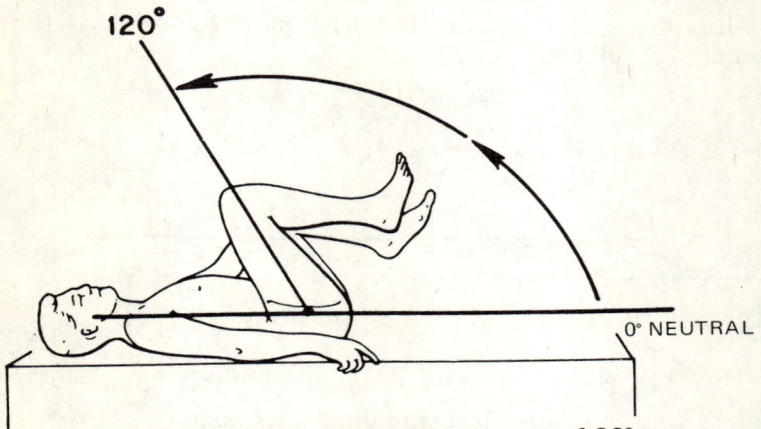

Fig. 79 Hip Flexion Contracture of 30°

The thigh and knee are now held with the hip flexed 90° and internal and external rotation are tested and recorded in degrees as shown in Figure 80.

ROTATION in FLEXION

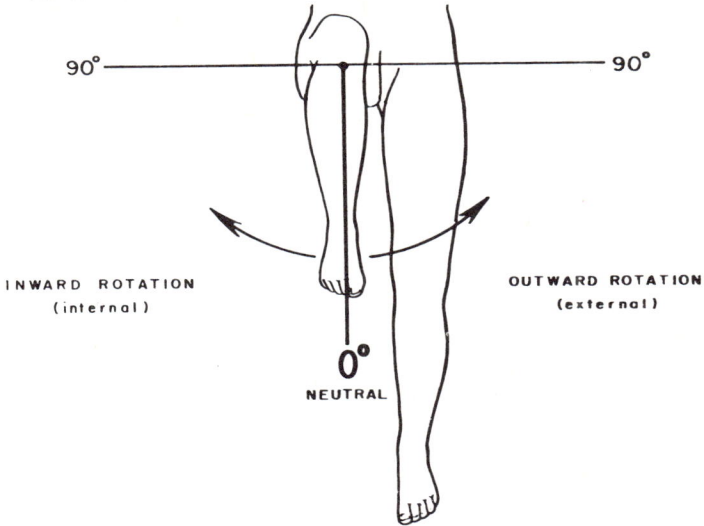

90° ————————————— 90°

INWARD ROTATION
(internal)

OUTWARD ROTATION
(external)

0°
NEUTRAL

Fig. 80 Limits Hip Rotation in Flexion

Rotation is also determined in extension in both the prone and supine position as shown in Figure 81.

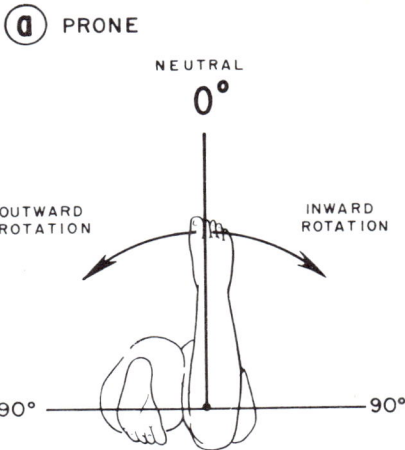

(a) PRONE

NEUTRAL
0°

OUTWARD
ROTATION

INWARD
ROTATION

90° ————— 90°

Fig. 81 (A) Hip Rotation in Extension—Prone

103

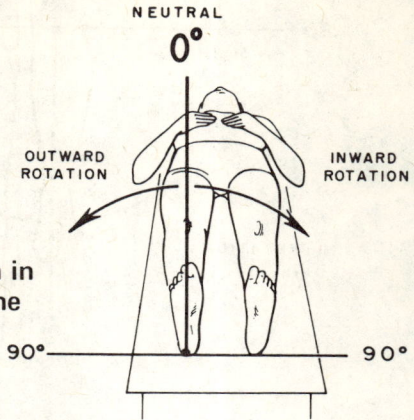

(b) SUPINE

NEUTRAL

0°

OUTWARD
ROTATION

INWARD
ROTATION

Fig. 81   (B) Hip Rotation in
Extension—Supine

90°   90°

Abduction and adduction of the hip are determined
in extension.

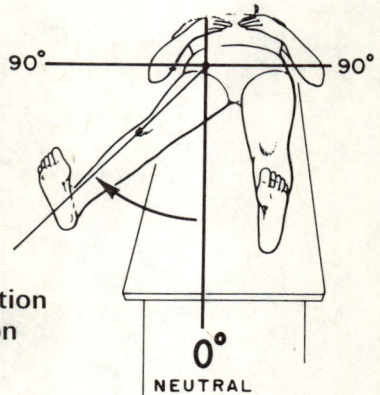

90°   90°

Fig. 82   Hip Abduction
in Extension

0°

NEUTRAL

The normal hip does not extend beyond the neutral
position. The limits of hip motion are shown by movements of the contralateral fixed hip as the normal ranges
of the observed hip are reached. It is well to remember
that in the standing position a hip flexion contracture may
be masked by an increased lumbar lordosis.

104

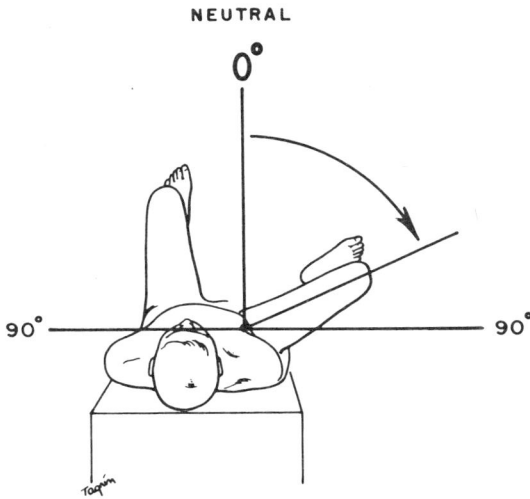

NEUTRAL

0°

90° — 90°

Fig. 83   Hip Abduction in Flexion

Abduction of the thigh is also determined with the hip flexed 90°.

Significant variation between abduction in flexion and extension indicates an abnormality of the hip.

The purpose of the examination of the range of motion of the hip joint is to identify clearly any restriction of normal motion. The findings will indicate either an acute or a chronic disease process. With an acute synovitis of the hip an effusion distends the capsule and physical examination reveals the lower extremity to be held in flexion, abduction, and external rotation. Testing for range of motion of such a joint will reveal a flexion contracture and loss of internal rotation. With a chronic synovitis of the hip joint the thigh is adducted, flexed and internally rotated. Testing the range of motion of such a hip joint reveals a flexion and adduction contracture, and limited flexion and rotation. As noted in the general physical examination, a fixed adduction contracture is frequently noted first as a functional shortening of the limb.

105

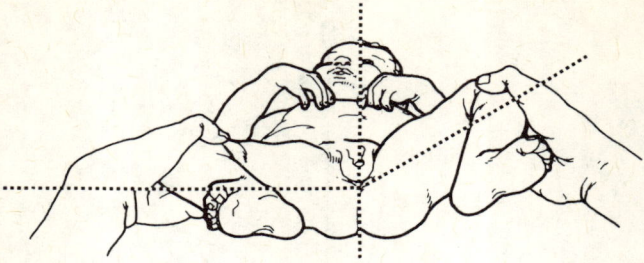

Fig. 84 Restricted abduction in congenital dislocation of the hip

One of the most common problems about the hip in infants and children is *congenital dislocation* of the *hip*. Part of the routine examination of the newborn is to examine for this abnormality. This is done as illustrated in Figure 84. The thighs of the child are placed in flexion and grasped so that the thumb of the examiner is against the knee and the examiner's fingers are placed firmly against the infants buttocks. In this position, gentle traction can be applied and the thighs abducted gently. Normally they should abduct 70° to 90°. If there is resistance to abduction on this test, a dislocation of the hip can be suspected. With gentle traction and abduction and with some pressure against the trochanters a "clunk" may be felt (*Ortelani's sign*). This is a strong indication that the infant has a congenitally dislocated hip. The "clunk" indicates the dislocated hip has been reduced and increased abduction may then be obtained.

The normal child standing on one foot stabilizes the pelvis against the pull of gravity by contracting the gluteus medius. The dislocated hip rides up decreasing the effectiveness of the gluteus medius allowing the opposite side of the pelvis to sag. This sag is known as the *Trendelenberg sign*. Such an unstable sag may be mitigated by tilting the trunk toward the affected hip. This position is known as a compensated Trendelenberg sign.

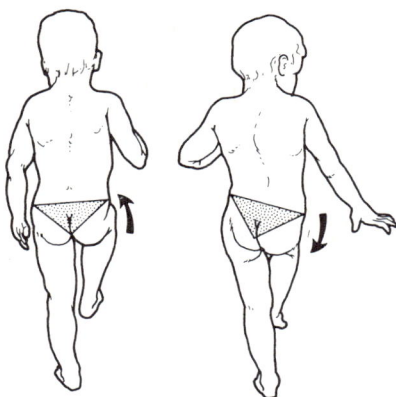

Fig. 85 Positive Trendelenberg Sign on the Right

In-toeing is a common complaint in children. Such a variation may be caused by *metatarsus adductus* of the foot or internal tibial torsion or both. These conditions have been described previously. Another cause of in-toeing in the child is increased anteversion of the neck of the femur. The normal anteversion angle is 15°-20°.

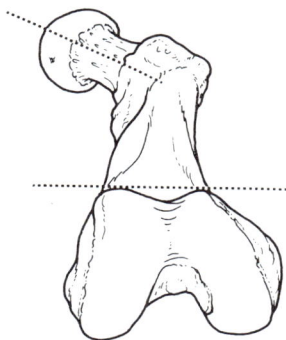

Fig. 86 Normal Anteversion of the femoral neck

An increase in the normal *anteversion* angle is reflected in the physical examination by an increased internal rotation of the hip. Normal internal rotation is 45°. The in-toeing child who has increased anteversion of the neck of the femur will demonstrate 60° to 90° of internal rotation. There is a corresponding decrease in external rotation. Therefore, neutral hip rotation for this child presents as internal rotation of the lower extremity.

The limit of normal adduction of the hips allows the thighs to cross at about the midshaft of the femur. When examining a child for adduction, if the thighs can be crossed at a higher level, one should suspect congenital deformity about the hip. The most common abnormalities causing such a finding is *proximal focal femoral deficiency* (absence) and severe coxa vara. In the standing position this is seen as flaring or widening of the hips.

Elderly patients are subject to an injury referred to as a *fractured hip,* actually a fracture of the proximal end of the femur. The patient presents with a shortened lower extremity that lies in more than the physiologic amount of external rotation.

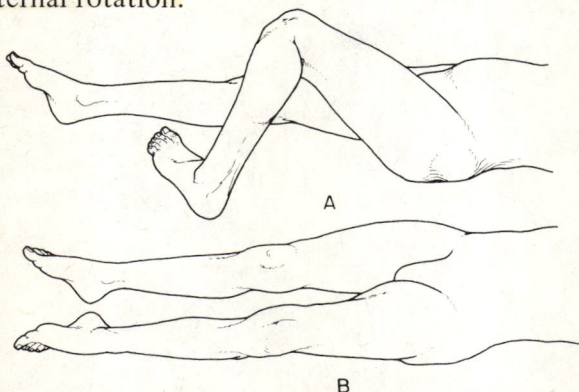

Fig. 87   A) Deformity of a posterior dislocation of the hip
B) Deformity of a fracture of the femoral neck

A fracture in the region of the femoral neck allows the large gluteal muscles to pull the shaft proximally and cause shortening. The weight of the limb externally rotates the lower extremity abnormally once the neck of the femur is broken. This is due, as previously noted, to the mass of the thigh being lateral to the center of hip motion. A patient with a fracture of the proximal femur will have moderate discomfort when the thigh is moved passively by the examiner.

The patient cannot voluntarily internally rotate the lower extremity. After adequate internal fixation of a fracture of the proximal femur the lower extremity will lie in its normal anatomic position. The observation that the patient can actively internally rotate the extremity and the absence of hip pain on passive motion further assure the stability of the fixation.

Younger patients suffer acute *dislocations* of the hip. This injury is usually inflicted when the hip is flexed in the sitting position and a severe force is directed against the knee. The femoral head dislocates posteriorly. Because the head of the femur is lying against the obliquity of the lateral wall of the pelvis, the thigh is flexed, internally rotated, and adducted. Examination of the hip reveals resistance to motion and severe pain.

In the normal gait the muscles about the hip play an important role in stabilizing the trunk and pelvis over the weight-bearing extremity. Weakness or paralysis of any of the major muscles results in a limp that is specific for the muscle involved.

Gluteus Medius Limp. When the patient stands on one extremity, the force of gravity pulls the torso and opposite extremity downwards. To counterbalance the pull of gravity, the gluteus medius must exert enough force to maintain the pelvis level (refer to general physical exam). When the gluteus medius muscle is paralyzed, the patient compensates for the lack of this counterbalancing muscle force by leaning the torso laterally over the involved hip joint as he advances the opposite lower extremity. This motion is done quickly and the resultant limp is called a "gluteus medius lurch." A "gluteus medius lurch" can also be caused by a painful hip. The strong contraction required of the gluteus medius to maintain stability irritates the hip and causes more pain. The patient decreases or eliminates the painful contraction of the muscle by lurching the torso toward the involved side.

Gluteus Maximus Limp. The gluteus maximus is important in maintaining the erect position of the torso. When standing, the spinal column is held upright by a balance of the muscles anterior and posterior to it. In walking, the torso is held in slight forward flexion. Paralysis of the gluteus maximus severely decreases the power of the supporting posterior muscles and the patient may fall. To avoid falling the patient balances his torso by extending the lumbar spine. If he extends too far, he can easily correct this by his normal anterior muscles. Walking with a sudden posterior lurch of the torso during stance phase is called a "gluteus maximum lurch." Considering these limps, one can appreciate that patients suffering localized paralysis at the hip must walk leaning into their weakness.

A gluteus maximus lurch may be seen in diseases of the hip joint as well.

Bony deformity about the hip may cause other characteristic limps. The patient with chronic *slipped capital femoral epiphysis* will walk with the involved extremity externally rotated. This is due to the anterior displacement of the neck of the femur on the femoral head.

The patient with osteoarthritis of the hip walks with a gluteus medius limp due to pain in the joint or atrophy of the gluteus medius muscle. The involved lower extremity is held in adduction, flexion and external rotation. An older patient, walking with a rather rolling gait, as the torso lurches from side to side, and with the lower extremities externally rotated and adducted, is typical of bilateral osteoarthritis of the hip. In the severest bilateral hip deformities in this disease, the adduction may be so severe that the extremities are crossed and during walking, one foot does not pass the other but rather comes to the other.

110

6. Spine and Pelvis

The central stabilizing structure of the back is the vertebral column, consisting of twenty-four individual bones placed upon the sacrum with its four segments fused in the adult and terminating caudally in the articulated coccyx. The complex muscular system of the back and of the entire trunk furnishes the dynamic support for the back. This system functions effectively only through its effect on the static supporting structures including the vertebral body with its component parts (centrum, processes, and articulations), the disc structures separating the vertebral bodies, and the numerous ligaments binding

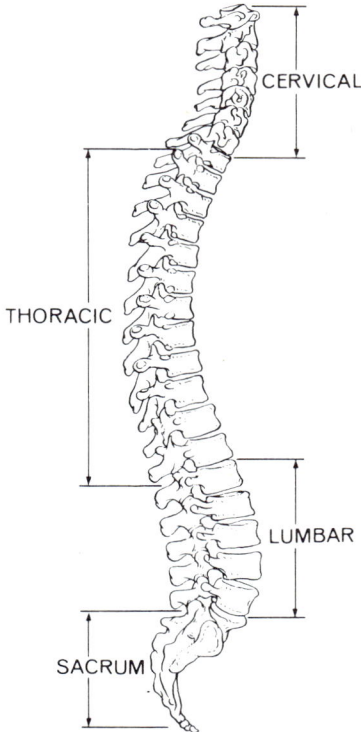

Fig. 88 Lateral view of the normal spinal curves

the individual parts into a functioning organ unit. These are the structures that are involved in any mechanical derangement of the back whether due to disease, injury or the aging process. With the cord and spinal roots in close approximation to these supporting structures, involvement of the nervous system may frequently accompany any derangement of the back. Any examination of the back must include assessment of these parts of the nervous system and any treatment program will always assign first priority to any involvement of the nervous system.

Measurement of standing height and sitting height is always a part of the examination of the back in a growing individual. For examination the back must be seen undraped with the individual standing. In the normal, there is lordosis in the cervical region, kyphosis in the thoracic region, and lordosis in the lumbar region; the head is aligned over the mid-line of the sacrum; and the shoulders are level. Any increase above the normal or decrease below the normal physiological curves is noted, as well as any deviation of the spine laterally. Sharp, angular deviation of the spine from the mid-line may be termed trunk list, or if occurring in the lumbar spine may be designated sciatic scoliosis. True scoliosis of the spine means lateral rotatory curvature with the aligning forces of the trunk, attempting, often unsuccessfully, to return the head to the midline.

Further inspection of the spine in general is carried on with the trunk bent forward in flexion. This is a particularly useful position in which to demonstrate rotation of some position of the spine. In the thoracic region, because of the accompanying rib deformity, even minor degrees of rotation may be noted. In the lumbar region rotation may be more difficult to outline.

Any abnormal pigmentation, dimpling, abnormal creasing, or abnormal hair concentration should be noted.

112

The range of motion of the various regions of the back is then noted, first in the standing position, and then in the sitting position. Motion in flexion-extension, in lateral bend to the left and to the right, and then in rotation to the left and to the right is noted. As spinal motion is represented by the sum of the motions at a number of joints rather than the motion at one, as in the hip or knee, one should note whether each segment is contributing its normal amount rather than look for a reduction in motion at one level and an increase at a level above or below.

Palpation of the spinal structures will often give additional information in the examination and may be used also to confirm information previously obtained by inspection and by observing movement.

Special maneuvers or tests designed to elicit specific information may be utilized when examining individual areas of the back.

As indicated previously, examination of the back will always include examination of those parts of the nervous system that may be involved in the area of the spine under review.

CERVICAL SPINE

Normally there is a lordosis of the cervical spine and the spinous processes of the seven cervical vertebrae are located exactly in the mid-line. Common deformities are: loss of the normal lordotic curve with the cervical spine flattened, lateral tilt of the head and the vertebrae to the right or to the left, or rotatory deformity with the face rotated to one side or to the other. The superior contours of both shoulders are noted in relation to the cervical spine. Some suggestion of soft tissue webbing between the neck and the shoulders may be seen with congential anomalies of the cervical vertebrae.

A) FLEXION and EXTENSION

NEUTRAL
0°

90°   90°

B) LATERAL BEND

NEUTRAL
0°

90°   90°

C) ROTATION

NEUTRAL
0°

90°   90°

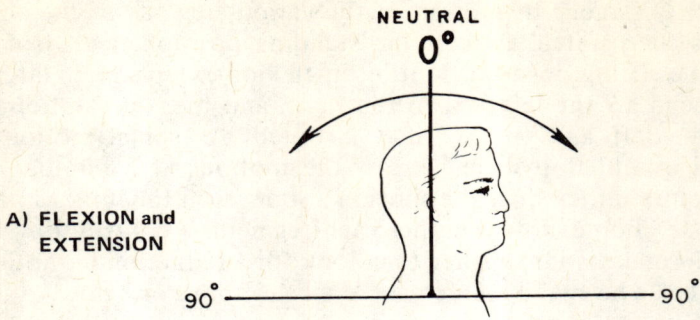

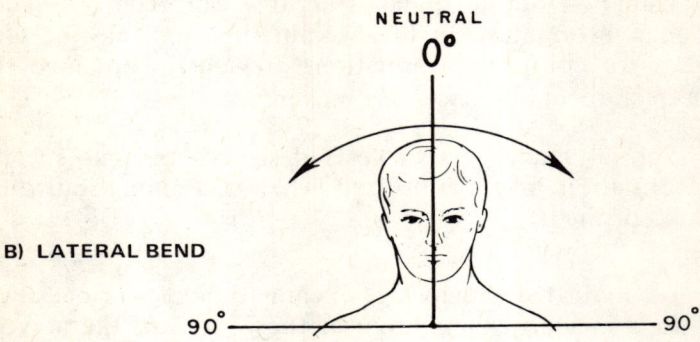

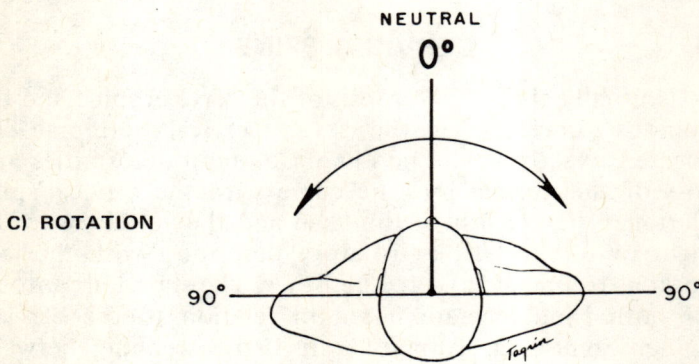

Fig. 89   Motions of the cervical spine

114

Palpation of the cervical spine is especially useful in distinguishing muscle spasm from contracture. With the latter, the soft tissues are rigid and unyielding while with spasm, although the muscles feel quite tight, there is some give beneath the examining finger. If abnormal position of the head and neck has been noted and if by palpation no contracture or spasm is detected, then one may suspect that the deformity may be in the bony structure of the neck, and this of course will be revealed by the roentgen examination.

Gentle palpation is always used to outline areas of tenderness and is particularly useful in an examination after injury. A fracture of any part of a vertebra is usually accompanied by local tenderness. In the cervical spine, palpation is used to determine the alignment of the spinous processes. Any derangement of the normal alignment may indicate vertebral displacement.

Motion in the cervical spine, as in all regions of the back, is complex and the total is the sum of small increments of motion at each of the vertebral joint levels. Flexion-extension in the normal is 80° to 90°, lateral bend is 60° to 70°, and rotation is 65° to 75°. Rotation takes place largely between C/1 and C/2 with lesser amounts at each of the other levels. The atlanto-occipital joint furnishes 15° to 25° of flexion with the remainder of the motion distributed somewhat evenly among the other intervertebral joints. Any measured restriction of motion may be due to muscle spasm resulting from injury either to the soft parts alone or to bone and joint structures as well. Restriction of motion may also be due to tight and shortened soft tissue structures, or it may be due to blockage by abnormal bony parts and frequently by a combination of the two. Degenerative disease of the cervical spine, seen in the adult, results in disc and bone distortion as well as soft tissue contracture with both of these factors contributing to the restriction of motion.

In some patients with degenerative disease, the additional factor of muscle spasm may further restrict cervical motion so that the true range of motion may not be appreciated until the muscle spasm has been completely relieved.

Neurological examination is always a part of the assessment of the cervical spine. As nervous system involvement in degenerative spondylosis is usually confined to the nerve roots, positive findings are thus confined to the upper extremities and a complete sensory, motor and reflex examination should be carried out. As degenerative change most commonly develops in the lower rather than the upper cervical spine, the nerve roots of C/5, C/6, C/7 or C/8 would be the ones likely to be involved. Atrophy, motor impairment, and reflex change in the triceps, the biceps, and brachialis will be noted in involvement of the upper portion of this spine segment and motor impairment in the muscles of the fingers will be noted in involvement in the lower portion of the segment. Sensory impairment will be found in the corresponding dermatomes, so that localization of the compression point causing symptoms and findings can usually be made to within one or two possible spinal levels. Less frequently degenerative changes in the cervical spine result in compression of the long tracts of the cord. In a typical case of this type, there will be motor and reflex impairment in one or both of the upper extremities, and hyperreflexia in one or both of the lower extremities with loss of the abdominal reflex.

Acute injury of the cervical spine involving bone or soft tissue either together or separately is more commonly noted at the C/4, C/5 level. When the nervous system is involved in injury at this level both spinal nerve roots and the cord are likely to be damaged. Careful neurological examination is required to place the level of the neurological involvement as this may often not correspond to the level of the bone, the joint, or the ligamentous injury.

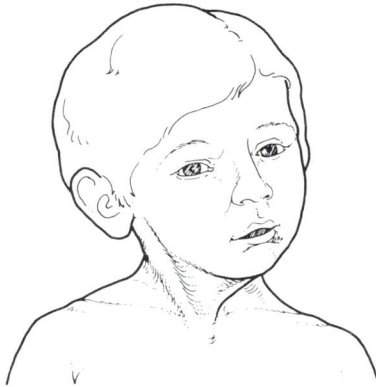

Fig. 90   Fixed deformity of Torticollis

A fixed lateral rotatory deformity of the cervical spine may at times be found in the young child and has been designated congenital torticollis. It is usually due to contracture of the sternocleidomastoid muscle that is easily recognized on inspection and palpation. Rotatory motion and lateral flexion in a direction opposite to that of the deformity will be restricted. The cause of this contracture of the sternocleidomastoideus is not known, but a soft tissue mass has been noted in the muscle in the newborn occasionally. Other causes of lateral rotatory deformity of the cervical spine are to be differentiated. Cervical hemivertebra or failure of vertebral segmentation may at times be the cause of such a deformity and ocular imbalance or unilateral eye disease may likewise be the cause of a somewhat similiar neck deformity.

THORACIC SPINE

The thoracic spine, due in part to the close attachment of the rib cage, is characterized by great stability and by limited mobility. Even in severe injury of this area of the spine, if the rib cage is spared, considerable stability of the vertebral structures persists. A small amount of motion in flexion-extension, in lateral bend, and in rotation is normally present with the amount largely dependent upon the mobility of the rib structures. Another feature of this area of the back is the early manifestation of any spine deformity by the magnified deformity of the thoracic cage. With lateral rotatory deformity of the thoracic spine, the involvement may be so slight as to pass unnoted in the spine itself, but because of the deforming rotatory force applied to the thorax, and the magnification of the rotation by the ribs, the deformity becomes quite obvious in the asymmetry of the chest wall.

As in all areas of the spine, inspection is an important part of the physical examination of the thoracic spine. Visible findings are noted and perhaps later reinforced by palpation and observation of motion. Spotty discoloration of the skin (cafe-au-lait) may alert the examiner to some underlying deformity as may abnormal distribution of hair, or unusual dimpling or contractures of the skin. The levels and symmetry of the shoulders are noted. Asymmetry may be due to lateral and rotatory deviation of the spine or it may be due to congenital elevation of one scapula (Sprengel's deformity). In this latter case a bone from the medial angle of the scapula to the seventh cervical vertebra may be palpated or instead a heavy fibrous band may be felt.

Prominence of the vertebral margin (winging) of the scapula indicates paresis or weakness of the serratus anterior muscle. Weakness of the trapezius of course, is indicated by dropping downward of the entire shoulder girdle.

Palpation of the thoracic spine may be used to reinforce the observations made by inspection, and is carried out with the patient standing and again with the patient in a prone position. The spinous processes are outlined to

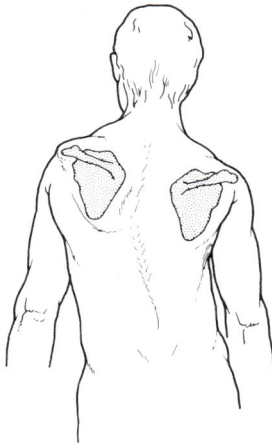

Fig. 91 High shoulder in Sprengel's Deformity

indicate their position in the mid-line or to denote any deviation from the mid-line. Separation of two adjacent spinous processes, in the axial plane, indicates some collapse of a vertebral body. In the lying position pressure over the spinous process or over a transverse process may elicit tenderness, indicating perhaps fracture or some other pathological change. Fracture of a rib is often more easily demonstrated by direct pressure than by x-ray and the ribs are always palpated for deformity as well as tenderness.

Although motion in the thoracic spine is limited by the thorax, some motion is demonstrated in flexion-extension, in lateral bend, and in rotation and thus should be carefully evaluated. Movement of the rib cage is closely related to spinal column movement and the inspiratory-expiratory excursion of the ribs should be carefully measured. In the adult it will usually be two inches or more. Severe restriction with excursion measuring less than one inch indicates restrictive spinal disease, probably ankylosing spondylitis.

119

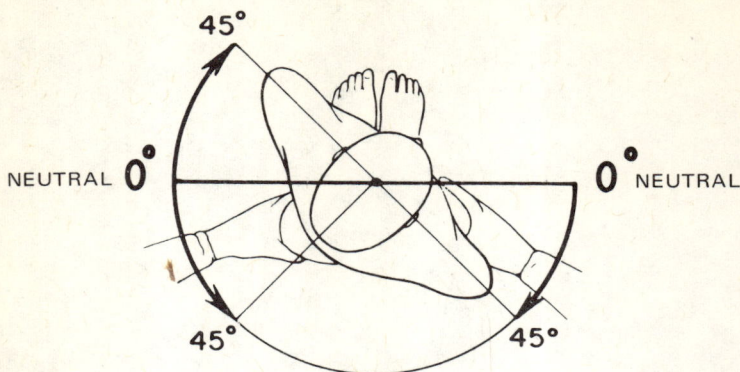

Fig. 92 Rotation of the spine

Scoliosis or lateral rotatory deformity of the spine in its more advanced form will involve the entire spine, but in its less severe form is usually seen in the thoracic spine. In its very mild form lateral deviation will not be accompanied by rotation, but because of the axis of movement between the vertebral bodies a limit to lateral deviation is soon reached beyond which lateral deviation can only proceed if accompanied by rotation. So that in even a moderate lateral curvature some amount of rotation is demonstrated. This is best done by having the patient bend forward. The distortion of the rib cage is immediately apparent and its severity can be noted. Scoliosis may be classified as postural or structural. In the former, the vertebral column assumes a laterally displaced position in the erect position, but when the prone position is assumed it disappears as there are no fixed structural elements to maintain the deformity after the effect of gravity is erased. In structural scoliosis the severity of the deformity may be reduced, but it is not completely corrected in the prone position because of the fixed deformity of the structural elements either in the soft tissues, in the bone structure, or more likely in both. If a corrective force is applied to the curvature either in an axial direction or laterally some

120

correction will usually be obtained and this may even be complete. During the examination some determination of the passive correctibility of the curve should be made by applying various forces.

In the presence of a lateral deformity of the vertebral column, the body will always attempt to maintain the head centered over the sacrum in the mid-line. This will result in secondary curves: one above the original or primary curvature and the other below the primary curve. Since these secondary curves form as the body attempts to compensate for the lateral trunk shift and maintain the head balanced in the mid-line, they may be termed compensatory curves as well as secondary curves. Secondary changes in the rib cage as well as the lateral and rotatory shift in the spine will commonly result in some imbalance in the shoulders and this may often be the presenting complaint. Likewise, any trunk shift will result in the prominence of the pelvis and hip either on the right or on the left. All of these features may be noted as the spine is inspected in the standing, sitting and lying positions.

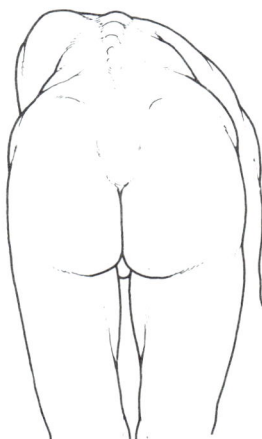

Fig. 93   Rotational deformity of Thoracic Scoliosis (seen in flexion)

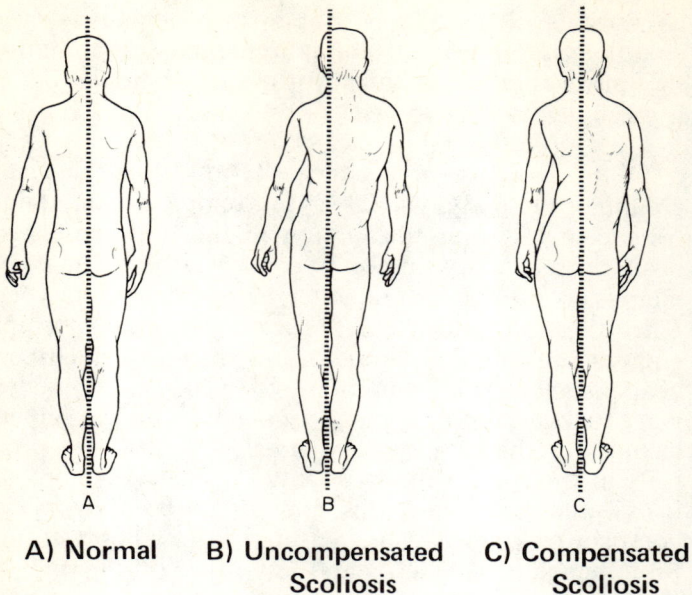

A) Normal   B) Uncompensated   C) Compensated
Scoliosis   Scoliosis

Fig. 94   Scoliosis

Bending motion is then noted in all of these positions and external force may be applied laterally and axially to note the flexibility of the curve. Standing and sitting heights are recorded and measurements of the lower lumbar curve are noted. As scoliosis may be produced by imbalance of the trunk muscles, all of these, including the abdominal muscles should be carefully tested for any weakness.

Increase in the normal anterior-posterior physiological curvature of the thoracic spine is called kyphosis. As in scoliosis this may be classified postural or structural. A postural kyphosis will show complete correction in the prone position while the structural type will show incomplete correction if any. This latter type may be caused by any disease, injury or congenital anomaly of the thoracic spine but in this country today is most commonly due to an affection of the vertebral growth centers, an osteochondritis that is known as Scheuermann's disease. The severity of the deformity resulting from this affection is dependent not only on the severity of the disease in the affected vertebral body and the subsequent wedging deformity, but also on the number of vertebrae involved and the level of these vertebrae in the spinal axis.

LUMBAR SPINE:

The lumbar spine is a much more flexible region of the back than the thoracic spine, especially in the anterior-posterior and the lateral planes. As it is the connecting link between the flexible trunk and the fixed platform of the pelvis it is likely to be subjected to large mechanical stresses. Low back pain is a common complaint in the population of today and it may be chronic or acute, each of which may be recurrent.

As in any other true joint of the body, the lumbo-sacral joint or any of the inter-lumbar joints may be strained with involvement of either capsule, ligament, or tendon, or more commonly, a combination of these — a lumbo-sacral strain. With the passage of time and continuation of the forces causing the strain certain of the structures may undergo pathological changes. Muscles and ligaments may be stretched and thinned, articular cartilage may be eroded in typical degenerative fashion, and hypertrophic bone changes may develop with encroachment on the neural canal or neural foramen. Early or late in the process the spinal posterior longitudinal ligament and anulus fibrosus may become attenuated, or may give way suddenly so that some of the nucleus pulposus pushes through the anulus fibrosus to bulge into the neural canal. With the roots of the cauda equina in close proximity, one or several of these may be compressed giving the clinical picture of sciatica. Or later, one of the roots, as it makes its exit through the foramen may be compressed by hypertrophic and inflammatory changes. This close proximity of neural structure to the supporting skeletal structures is an important consideration in the examination of the lumbar spine and no examination of this region of the spine is complete without a full examination of the neural structures that may be involved.

Inspection of the lumbar region will disclose any of the cutaneous abnormalities that have been described in the other sections of the spine. In the normal individual the lumbar spine assumes a mildly lordotic position in the sagittal plane and of course, does not deviate to the right or left. As a sign of disease or injury, the lordotic position may be completely lost and this normal curve reversed. The spine may be shifted to the right or to the left. This may often be a manifestation of a protruded disc and the imposed sciatic pain and has been termed sciatic scoliosis. Either the flattening or the list to the right or left or both of them together is the result of lumbar muscle spasm.

Palpation, best carried out with the patient in a prone position, is performed to assess the presence or absence of spasm, locate points of tenderness and determine the alignment of the lumbar spinous processes. Following injury one or several of these may be displaced to one side or the other or they may be irregularly spaced longitudinally. Palpation may also be used to examine the transverse processes. Scoliosis in the lumbar spine, as in the thoracic spine, exhibits vertebral rotation as well as lateral displacement. In the thoracic spine the deformity is exaggerated in the rib cage and is quickly recognized. In the lumbar spine a similar degree of rotation may be present, but less obvious. Palpation along the levels of the transverse processes may give some indication of this deformity that otherwise might pass unnoted. Palpation eliciting pain localized over a transverse process is useful in indicating a fracture of that part following injury.

Motion is then observed. As in other parts of the spine, the motion observed in the lumbar spine is the sum of the motions at the individual intervertebral lumbar joints. Because of the proximity of the hip joints, the examiner must take care to establish that the motion is in the lumbar spine and not the hip joint. A useful method is to grasp the pelvis by spanning it with both hands while the patient moves the spine in the desired direction. Any coincidental motion through the hips will then be evident as the pelvis moves.

Motions described in the examination are flexion, extension, bend to the right and bend to the left. Motion may be recorded as the percentage of motion expected in the normal individual or specific measurements may be given. In the motion of flexion of the spine the axis of rotation of the vertebrae lies anterior to the spinous processes. During flexion, the distance between adjacent spinous processes gradually increases and then as the spine is extended the spinous processes are brought closer together. Using a tape measure the examiner can thus measure the total distance of the excursion of the spine in flexion and extension. As trunk motion may be affected by spasm of the hamstring group, it is always observed with the patient standing and then with the patient sitting when the hamstrings are completely relaxed. Restriction of motion in the spine, as is true in all joints of the body, may be due to deformity of the bone structure, to contracture of the soft tissues, including tendon, ligament, or muscle, or to spasm of the spinal muscles. This latter is determined largely by palpation of the spinal muscle masses. Restriction of motion may frequently be the result of all of these factors with the additional factor of pain further restricting the arc of motion. Any pain elicited by motion should be described indicating its location and the motion producing it.

The straight leg raising or Lasegue test is performed with the patient lying in a supine position. The limb to be

125

tested is grasped behind the ankle and the extremity is then brought up passively into hip flexion with the knee maintained in full extension. This maneuver stretches the sciatic nerve as it curves around the hip joint and relaxation of the nerve by flexion of the knee is not permitted. If one or several of the nerve roots has already been stretched or irritated within the vertebral canal by protruded disc or osteophyte, continuance of the test motion will cause marked increase in pain and the examiner will be forced to stop. This point is noted as the level of the straight leg raising sign. In the normal, the straight leg can usually be brought to a full 90°. If on reaching the point of pain production, the examiner then lowers the extremity a few degrees, he may then again elicit sharp pain by passively dorsi-flexing the ankle. This is termed the Lasegue sign and is simply another method of applying further stretch to the irritated sciatic nerve. Considerable care and experience are necessary in interpreting the straight leg raising sign. Some individuals have tight hamstring and other muscles. In others the hamstrings may be in spasm from injury or other cause so that the straight leg raising maneuver may be restricted in the absence of sciatic irritation. It is often useful to utilize a variation of the usual procedure in performing the straight leg raising sign by having the patient sit over the edge of the examining table with the knees flexed. The examiner then passively extends the knee. Under the usual circumstances of a positive test the patient immediately attempts to extend the hips by moving the trunk backward. Usually in doing this the patient will support the trunk with the extended upper extremities showing what has been called the tripod sign. This second form of the test procedure may be carried out in an informal and casual manner during the examination of the lower extremity reflexes and may be useful in establishing whether the test as carried out in the supine position was really a false positive response.

The lumbo-sacral joint, a term which we take to include the fourth lumbar joint as well as the fifth lumbo-sacral joint, is one of the most frequently injured joints of the body. The injury may be acute and instantaneous as when this level of the back is strained in lifting a heavy object, or it may be chronic with disability the result of a summation of a long series of incidents of minor strain. A history of improvement and then recurrence is quite common. The strain may often involve only the ligamentous structures about these joints, but at other times, the posterior longitudinal ligament may be stretched or torn allowing some of the intervertebral disc (the nucleus pulpuses, anulus fibrosus or both of these elements) to impinge or herniate into the vertebral canal. If this happens, because of the proximity of the lumbar and sacral nerve roots, one or several of these roots will quite likely be compressed giving the picture of a protruded lumbar disc. As the most frequently encountered level of the protrusion is the fourth lumbar-fifth lumbar or the fifth lumbar-first sacral level, the roots most likely to be involved are the fifth lumbar and the first sacral or not uncommonly, both, usually on only one side of the body.

The history given by the patient suffering from such a disability may be one of short duration with the onset associated with recent injury, or one of long duration with episodes of improvement and recurrence over a long period of time. On inspection the examiner may note that the patient's trunk is shifted sharply to the right or to the left and that the usual lumbar lordosis is obliterated. By palpation it will be evident that the para-spinal muscles are quite tense, protecting the spine against any movement. Further palpation with the patient in a prone position may elicit tenderness as the spinous process of L/5 or of L/4 is firmly pressed. Tenderness may be further elicited by pressure over the sciatic nerve as it emerges from the sacro-sciatic notch or further along its course in the posterior thigh. Motion throughout the lumbar spine, with the patient either standing or sitting may be completely obliterated, with the trunk rigid and moving only by motion at the hip joints. If any small amount of motion is present, extension is likely to produce a sudden increase in the intensity of the pain.

The straight leg raising test will usually be positive on the involved side after the extremity is flexed perhaps only a few degrees. The Lasegue sign will likewise give a strongly positive response.

A careful neurological evaluation may further define the pathological changes responsible for the complaints and disability. Careful circumferential measurements of the thighs and of the calves are made with the involved side often showing some atrophy. Sensation is then carefully tested using touch, pin prick and vibration stimuli. As the most common site of intervertebral disc protrusion is at the L/4-L/5 or the L/5-S/1 level, the most common area of sensory impairment will be the inner side or the outer side of the foot. Muscle strength is then tested throughout the lower extremities. Although some weakness as well as some atrophy may be noted in the gluteal muscles, weakness is most commonly demonstrated in the dorsi-flexors of the foot including the toe extensors. Reflexes are next tested and the Achilles reflex may be depressed or absent as the result of root compression from an intervertebral disc protruded at the L/5-S/1 interspace.

The sacrum, consisting of five fused vertebrae is relatively superficial and is examined directly. Any mass protruding dorsally is easily palpable and any fracture is usually demonstrated by eliciting sharply localized tenderness over the fracture line. The two sacro-iliac joints are large, stable, and resistant to any but severe trauma because of the bone structure itself, the deep placement of the joints, and the heavy ligamentous structure surrounding them. One or both joints may be involved by disease such as infection or may be separated by severe injury to the pelvic ring. Separation of one or both may occur in association with separation of the symphysis pubis during childbirth. Injury or disease may be indicated by local

128

tenderness to direct pressure over the joint, by pain produced over the joint as the iliac wings are compressed, or by localized pain produced by exerting torsional stress across the joint as one hip is hyperflexed and the other is hyperextended.

The coccyx is attached to the sacrum through the movable sacrococcygeal joint. This joint may be the site of painful osteoarthritis, and it may be injured in a fall directly upon it. The coccyx may be palpated directly over the posterior surface, and through the rectum over the anterior surface so that any displacement of the bone or any abnormal mobility is thus easily determined.

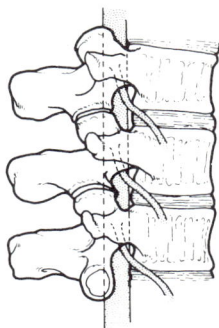

Fig. 95 **Lumbar Vertebrate, Disc, and Nerve Roots (lateral view)**

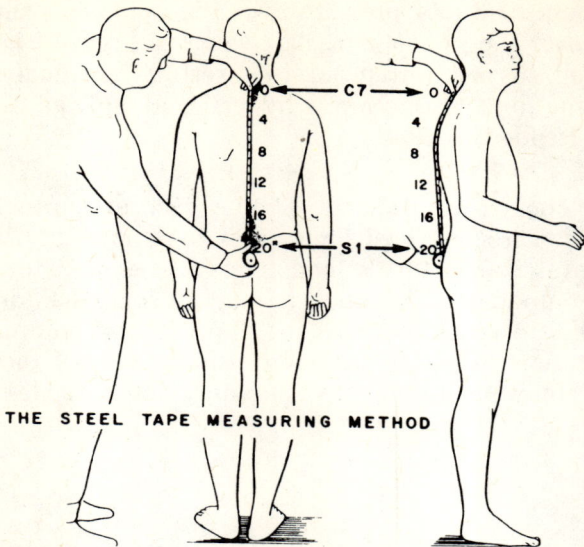

THE STEEL TAPE MEASURING METHOD

Fig. A THE PATIENT STANDING ERECT

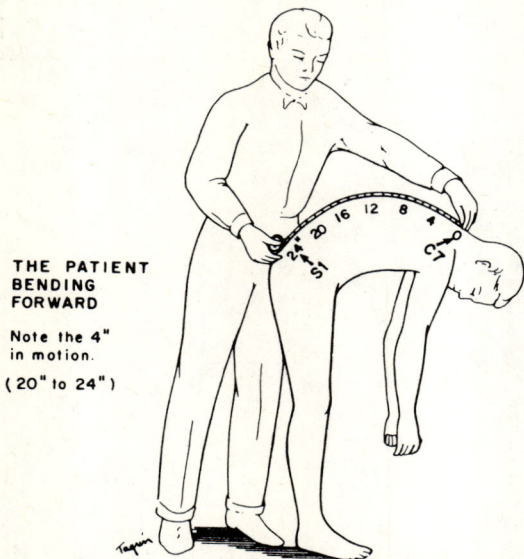

THE PATIENT
BENDING
FORWARD

Note the 4"
in motion.

(20" to 24")

Fig. 96 Measuring spinal flexion

130

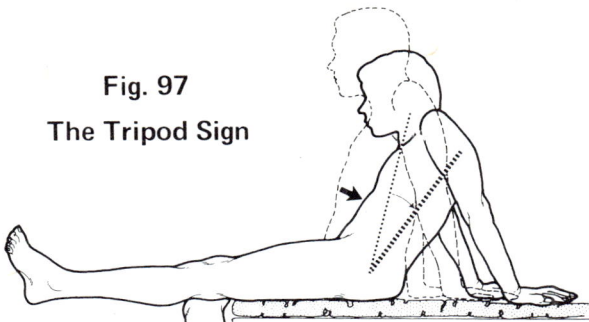

Fig. 97
The Tripod Sign

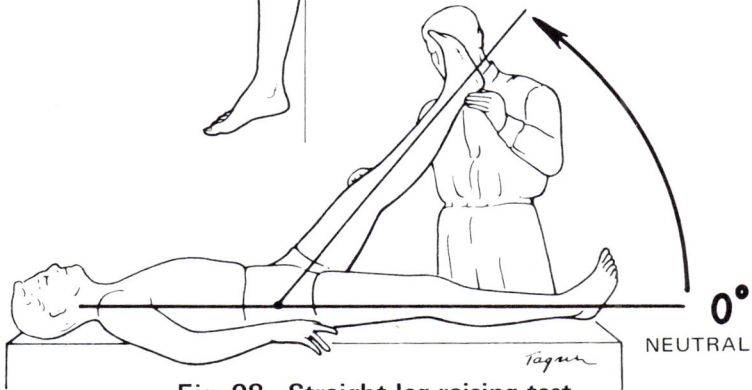

0°
NEUTRAL

Fig. 98   Straight leg raising test

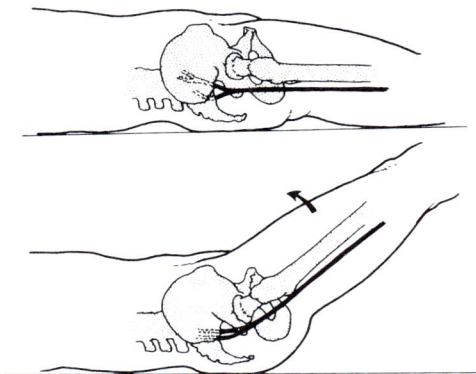

Fig. 99   Sciatic tension caused by straight leg raising

7. Shoulder and Arm

UPPER EXTREMITY: Shoulder and Arm

The shoulder joint is a compound joint, consisting of component parts, the glenohumeral joint, the acromio-clavicular joint, the sterno-clavicular joint, and the rotatory sliding movement of the scapula on the thorax, functioning as a joint. Examination must include each of these parts and then the units as a functioning whole.

The examination is carried out with the patient standing, sitting and lying. The prominent landmark, the acro-

GLOBAL MOTION of the SHOULDER

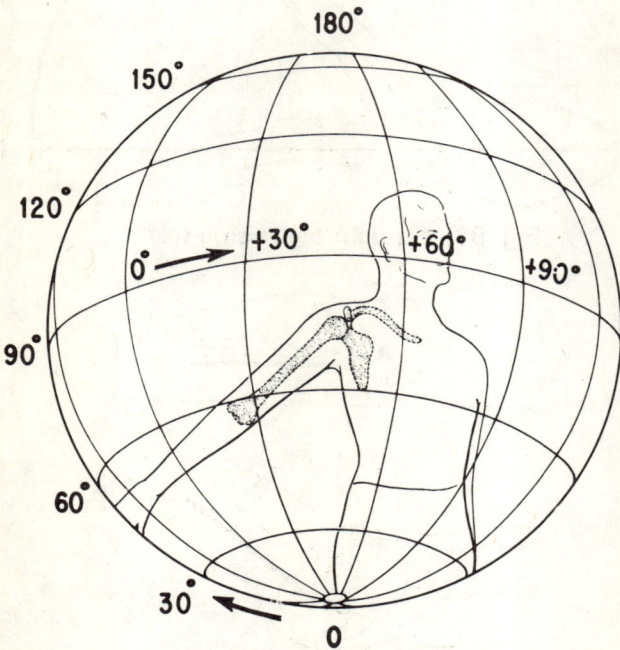

Fig. 100 Shoulder motion

mion process lying laterally and subcutaneously is easily noted even in the obese individual. Also lying subcutaneously and likewise easily palpable is the clavicle and the spine of the scapula, both useful in outlining the boundaries of this joint. Any displacement of any or several of these parts should be readily noted on inspection and palpation and by comparing with the opposite shoulder.

The clavicle and spine of the scapula are also subcutaneous for ready visibility and palpation. By looking and feeling, any displacement of the component elements may be determined by comparison to the opposite normal side.

A *"shoulder separation"* occurs at the acromio-clavicular joint. The clavicle appears to ride higher than the normal anatomical position and with pressure may be forced back into its normal position. It may likewise be moved forward and backwards from its elevated position indicating that not only has the joint capsule been ruptured but also the accessory coraco-clavicular ligament has been torn.

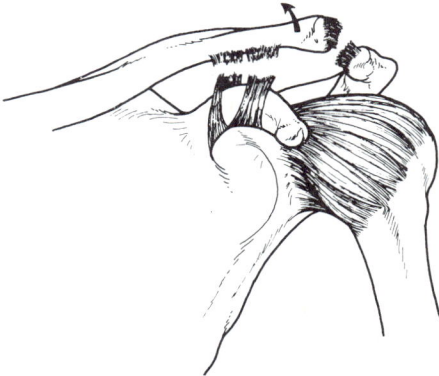

Fig. 101   Acromo-clavicular separation

Inspection and palpation will also disclose any break or deformity along the clavicle or alteration at the sternoclavicular joint.

133

In the normal shoulder, the smoothly rounded contours of the humeral head are seen below the acromion and any displacement of the head from the glenoid fossa can be noted by the flattening or indentation of this contour. *Dislocation of the humeral head* from the glenoid fossa occurs usually in an anterior direction with the head finally resting below the coracoid process. The patient with this injury often appears with the forearm of the affected extremity carefully supported by the uninjured extremity in a position of internal rotation. In addition to noting the altered convex contour of the shoulder, palpation will reveal the disappearance of the humeral head from beneath the acromion while palpation over the pectoralis muscle just below the coracoid process will demonstrate the firm humeral head lying in this position.

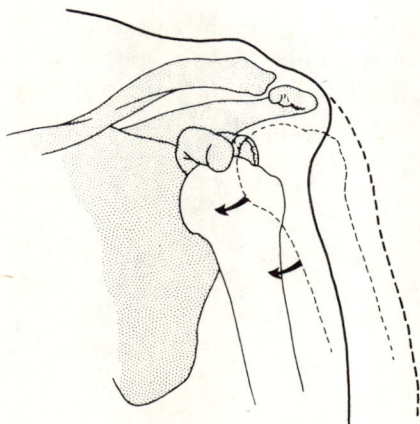

Fig. 102   Position of anterior dislocated shoulder

Less frequently the humeral head may displace posteriorly lying either at the edge of the glenoid or at the base of the scapular spine. In this case, the arm will not be restricted to the side in internal rotation and inability to internally rotate the extremity will suggest the diagnosis. Examination of both shoulder joints from above with the patient seated will demonstrate by inspection and palpation the loss of the rounded contours lateral to and anterior to the acromion process and a fullness posterior to it.

At times, swelling of the subacromial bursa may be noted by inspection and palpation of the area. Swelling of the glenohumeral joint capsule and atrophy of the shoulder muscles are best appreciated with the patient placed in a seated position. Viewed from above, any swelling or atrophy may be noted by comparison with the normal side.

Palpation may reveal points of tenderness, especially noted in acute *tendinitis* with calcification in one of the tendons comprising the tendinous cuff of this joint. This well-localized area of tenderness is most commonly noted in the supraspinatus tendon just below the tip of the acromion.

Motion at the shoulder joint is the resultant of motion occurring in the four component joints and, in the normal subject as the arm is raised overhead from the side, is spoken of as thoracic scapulo-humeral rhythm. All of the many muscles attached to the bones comprising the articulation partake in any movement by contracting or relaxing to produce the balanced rhythmic motion. In abduction in the neutral position, during the first 30° of motion, the scapula is moved into a position of stability by the muscles attached to this bone and the trunk. At the same time the scapulo-humeral muscles fix the humeral head in the glenoid cavity and initiate glenohumeral abduction. From this point as the arm is raised further into abduction, both glenohumeral and scapulothoracic motion contribute to the total abduction in a ratio of about 2 to 1 until the full 180° of abduction is accomplished. Any break in this balanced rhythm is indicative of some abnormality in one of the joints or in some part of the motor system. If disease or injury results in the complete freezing of glenohumeral motion, the movement of the scapula on the thorax will permit the arm to be raised about 90° from the side although the normal rhythm will be lost.

Forward flexion and backward extension of the shoulder girdle are measured in degrees from the neutral starting position. This is primary motion of the scapula and the clavicle.

Upward motion of the shoulder girdle in elevation is measured in degrees. The opposite downward motion may be described as "depression" of the shoulder. Rotatory motion in the shoulder girdle is possible but cannot be accurately measured. It can be estimated in percentage of motion as compared to individuals of similar age and physique.

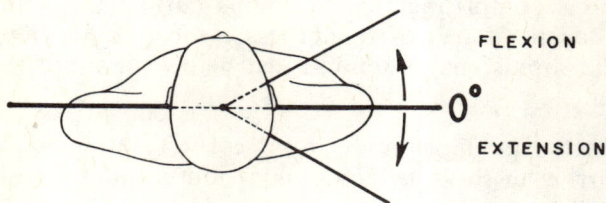

FLEXION

0°

EXTENSION

Fig. A

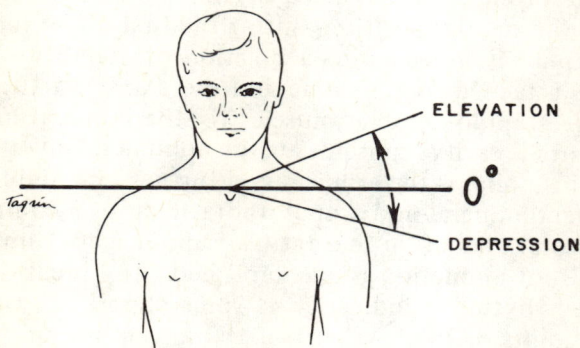

ELEVATION

0°

DEPRESSION

Fig. B

Fig. 103 Shoulder motions

The total upward motion of the arm at the shoulder from zero degrees to 180° is a smooth, rhythmic combination of true glenohumeral motion, plus the upward and forward rotation of the scapula on the chest wall with elevation of the clavicle and some rotation of this bone on its longitudinal axis. This motion is best noted with the patient in the standing position.

Zero Starting Position: The patient standing erect, with the arm at the side of the body.

1. Vertical or upward motion of the shoulder.

Abduction is the upward motion of the arm away from the side of the body in the coronal plane, from 0° to 180°. Adduction is the opposite motion of the arm toward the midline of the body, or beyond it in an upward direction.

Forward flexion is the forward upward motion of the arm in the anterior sagittal plane of the body, from 0° to 180°. The opposite motion to the zero position may be termed "depression" of the arm.

Backward extension is the upward motion of the arm in the sagittal plane posterior to the body.

2. Horizontal motion of the shoulder. Horizontal flexion is the motion of the arm in the horizontal plane anterior to the coronal plane across the body.

Horizontal extension is the horizontal motion posterior to the coronal plane of the body.

Terminology identifying upward motion of the arm at the shoulder in various horizontal positions. This motion can take place between positions G and C in Figure 105.

Position A

Neutral Abduction: This is the upward motion of the arm from the side of the body from 0° to 180° in the coronal plane.

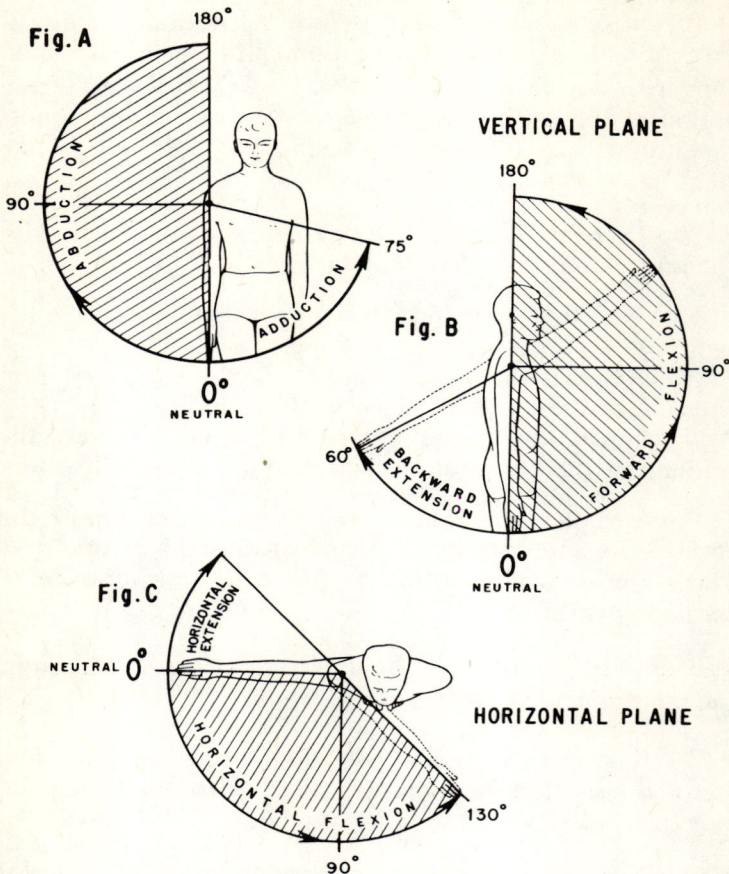

Fig. A

180°

ABDUCTION

90°

ADDUCTION

75°

0°
NEUTRAL

VERTICAL PLANE

180°

FLEXION

90°

Fig. B

BACKWARD EXTENSION

60°

FORWARD FLEXION

0°
NEUTRAL

Fig. C

HORIZONTAL EXTENSION

NEUTRAL 0°

HORIZONTAL FLEXION

HORIZONTAL PLANE

130°

90°

Fig. 104   Shoulder motions

Position B

The upward motion of the arm (abduction) in this position is taking place at 45° of horizontal flexion. If the upward motion at this position is 90°, then we describe this as "90° of abduction at 45° of horizontal flexion." This accurately defines the position of the extremity in two planes—the vertical (abduction) and the horizontal (flexion).

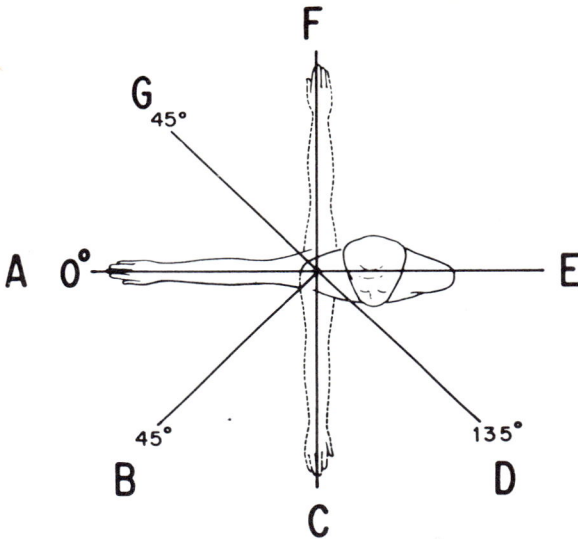

POSITION A = Neutral abduction

B = Abduction in 45° of horizontal flexion

C = Forward flexion

D = Adduction in 135° of horizontal flexion

E = Neutral adduction

F = Backward extension

G = Abduction in 45° of horizontal extension

Fig. 105 Shoulder motions

Position C

Upward or vertical motion of the arm directly in front of the body is described as forward flexion (from 0° to 180°).

Position D

Upward motion of the arm in this position is adduction of the arm upward at 135° of horizontal flexion.

139

Position E

Neutral adduction of the arm in the coronal plane.

Position F

Backward extension of the arm the sagittal plane.

Position G

Upward motion at this position is abduction of the arm, at 45° of horizontal extension.

Rotation

Neutral Position

It is customary to measure rotation of the shoulders in two positions: with the arm at the side of the body and in 90° of abduction. Rotation can also be measured in any position in which planes or coordinates are defined.

Rotation with arm at side of body

Inward and outward rotation is recorded in degrees of motion from the neutral starting point.

Rotation in abduction

Rotation in this position is less than with the arm at the side of the body. It is recorded in degrees of motion from the zero starting point.

A clinical method of estimating rotation is the distance the fingertips reach in relation to the scapula (internal rotation) or the base of the neck (external rotation).

Restriction of rotation with the arm at the side of the body may be found in a "*frozen shoulder*" or in *tendinitis* involving the subscapularis. In acute subacromial bursitis, if this motion is tested gently, little restriction may be noted. However, if the arm is taken into some abduction, the attempt to demonstrate external rotation will be resisted.

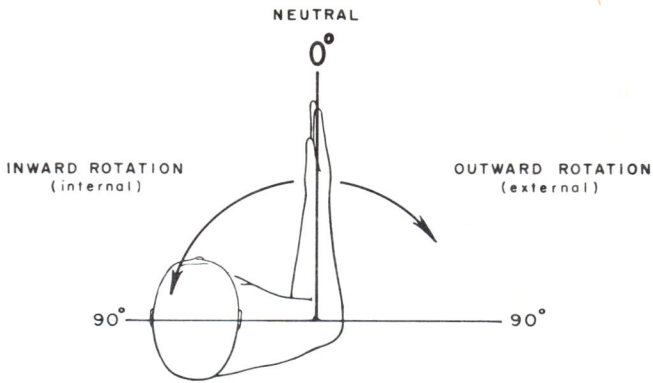

Fig. A   ROTATION WITH ARM AT SIDE

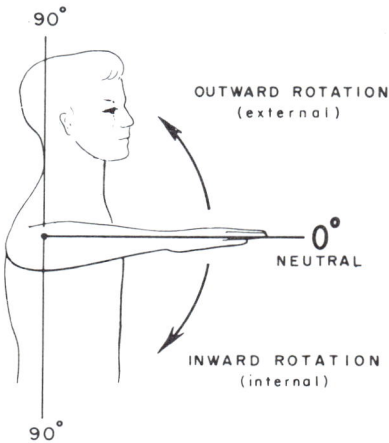

Fig. B ROTATION IN ABDUCTION

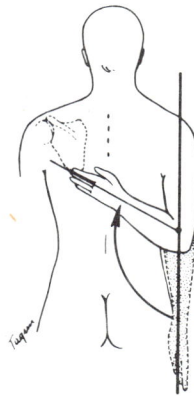

Fig. C
INTERNAL ROTATION
POSTERIORLY

Fig. 106 Rotary shoulder motion

141

Glenohumeral motion

It is important to differentiate true glenohumeral motion as opposed to scapulothoracic motion. The total upward motion of the arm at the shoulder from 0° to 180° is a smooth rhythmic combination of true glenohumeral

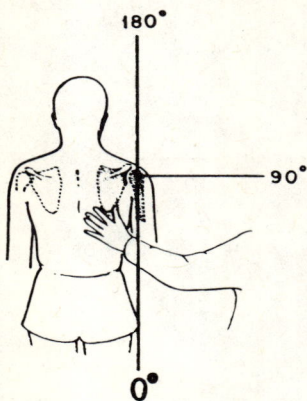

Fig. A NEUTRAL

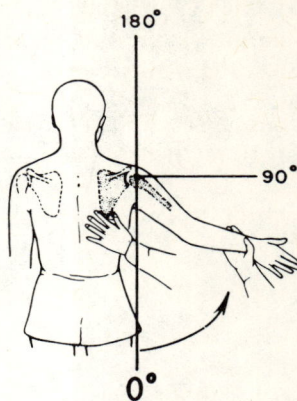

Fig. B RANGE OF TRUE GLENOHUMERAL MOTION

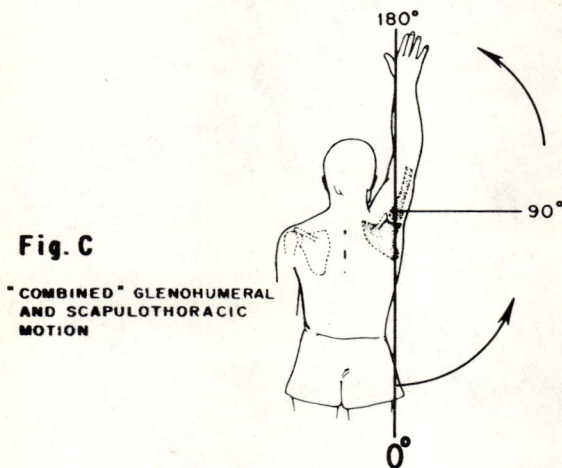

Fig. C

"COMBINED" GLENOHUMERAL AND SCAPULOTHORACIC MOTION

Fig. 107   Glenohumeral and scapulothoracic motion

motion, plus the upward and forward rotation of the scapula on the chest wall, or scapulothoracic motion.

The neutral starting position is with the arm at the side of the body.

True glenohumeral motion is estimted by fixing the scapula with one hand, and elevating the arm passively with the other hand.

In "combined" glenohumeral and scapulothoracic motion the rotation of the scapula upward and forward over the chest wall allows the arm to reach further upwards. Normally, the range is 180°.

MUSCLE PARALYSIS

Partial or complete paralysis of one or several of the muscles of the shoulder may be seen at times following injury that has resulted in interruption of one of the nerves supplying those muscles. Deltoid weakness or paralysis following dislocation of the humeral head is indicative of axillary nerve interruption. *Deltoid paralysis* is manifested by inability to maintain 90° of abduction against gravity. Paralysis of the serratus anterior muscle may follow compression of the long thoracic nerve by a tight binding in the axilla or by a sharp blow in that area. This may be demonstrated by *winging of the scapula.* Paralysis of the trapezius may result from injury to the spinal accessory nerve in the neck and is indicated by inability to shrug the shoulder.

Rupture of one or several of the short rotator muscles in the shoulder, usually the supraspinatus and/or the infraspinatus, may be indicated by the loss of ability to initiate abduction or by inability to maintain abduction against resistance because of weakness or pain. At times in a thinly muscled individual, the defect in the tendon may be felt.

8. Elbow and Forearm

The elbow is a hinge joint with the humerus and its two articular processes, the trochlea and the capitulum, furnishing one side of the hinge and matching the opposite side furnished by the olecranon process, the greater sigmoid notch of the ulna and the concave articular surface of the radial head. The osseous configuration of the joint provides strong stability that is further reinforced by the medial and lateral ligaments, the joint capsule and the muscles traversing the joint.

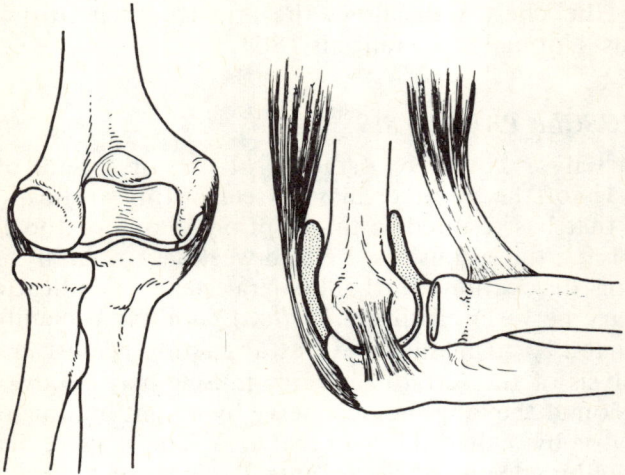

Fig. 108   Anatomy of the Elbow

The landmarks of this joint are the medial and lateral epicondyles of the humerus and the olecranon process of the ulna. The relationships of these three points should be noted with the elbow flexed to 90° when they form an equilateral triangle and with the elbow extended when the relationship is noted as a straight line. A common *elbow* injury is that of *posterior dislocation*. On examination of a patient with this injury, the olecranon is found displaced posteriorly with the normal triangular relationship disturbed. Another injury frequently encountered, especially in children, is that of *supracondylar fracture.*

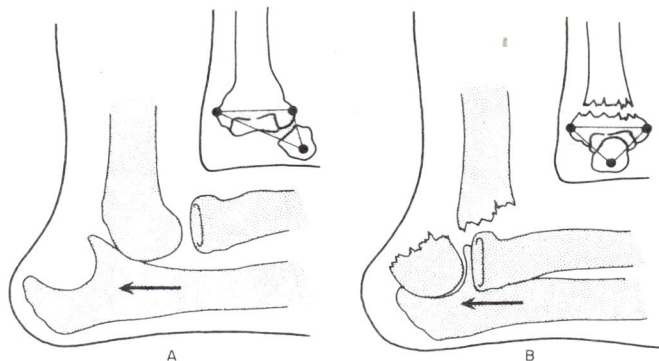

Fig. 109   Bony landmarks of the elbow in
A) Posterior dislocation
B) Supracondylar fracture

In this case, the bulge of the olecranon posteriorly may again be noted but as the epicondyles have been similarly displaced, the normal triangular relationship is preserved.

Fractures at the lower end of the humerus may frequently result in lateral deformity of the elbow as the result of faulty reduction or immobilization or as the result of epiphyseal injury. It is noted that the relationship of the extended supinated forearm to the arm is not a straight line but in the normal is represented by an angulation of the forearm lateralward of 15°, denoting the "*carrying angle.*" If this angle is greater than 15° the deformity is termed *cubitus valgus* and if less or reversed it is termed *cubitus varus.*

Because of the proximity of the brachial artery, and the radial, median, and ulnar nerves to the elbow joint, injuries

145

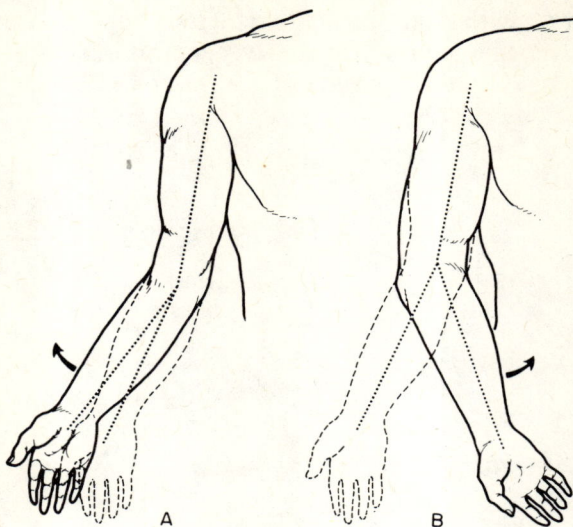

Fig. 110 Deformed "carrying angle"
A) Valgus B) Varus

of this region demand careful examination for evidence of any injury to these structures. With severe trauma about the elbow, it is mandatory to record the presence or absence of signs indicative of nerve or vessel injury. A person with cubitus valgus may some years following the original injury develop ulnar nerve palsy with the peripheral signs of this neuropathy demonstrable as well as tenderness and irritability of the nerve as it is palpated in its groove behind the medial condyle.

Distension of the joint by fluid is best appreciated by palpation over the postero-lateral portion of the joint between the lateral epicondyle and the radial head. This is most commonly seen when the joint is distended by the blood escaping from a fracture of the radial head. This injury is also indicated by well-localized tenderness over the head.

146

The olecranon bursa may be irritated by chronic repeated pressure injury or by a sudden direct blow with resultant swelling due to fluid or blood in the bursa. The diagnosis of such involvement is readily made since the bursa is subcutaneous.

In young children, strong extension of the elbow by an older individual may result in inability of the child to flex the elbow. Rotation of the forearm into supination and slight flexion usually results in a palpable jog with the elbow activated easily thereafter *(Nursemaid's elbow)*.

Motions

The natural motion is flexion. The opposite motion to flexion as far as the zero starting position is extension.

Any motion beyond the zero starting position is unnatural and is referred to as *hyperextension.*

Extension: 150° to 0° (from the angle of greatest flexion to the 0° position).

Hyperextension: This is measured in degrees beyond the zero starting point. This motion is not present in all individuals. When it is present, it may vary from 5° to 15°.

Measurement of Limited Motion

(The unshaded area in Figure 111 indicates the range of limited motion).

Limited motion may be expressed in the following ways:

(1) The elbow flexes from 30° to 90° (30 - 90).

(2) The elbow has a flexion deformity of 30° with further flexion to 90°.

As the ulna is subcutaneous throughout its length, it is easily palpable and any break in its continuity may be noted. The radius is less readily accessible but is palpable throughout its distal half. The motions of pronation and supination are rotary motions of the forearm that

147

result from the motion between the radius and ulna that takes place at the proximal and distal radialulnar joints. Disturbances at these joints are the most common causes of restriction of forearm pronation and supination.

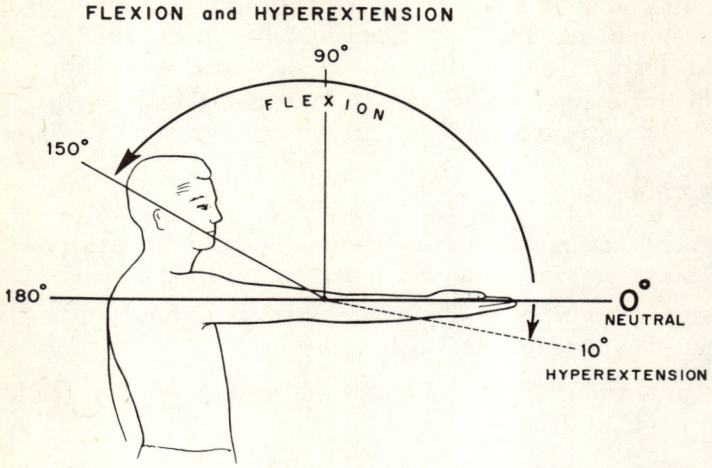

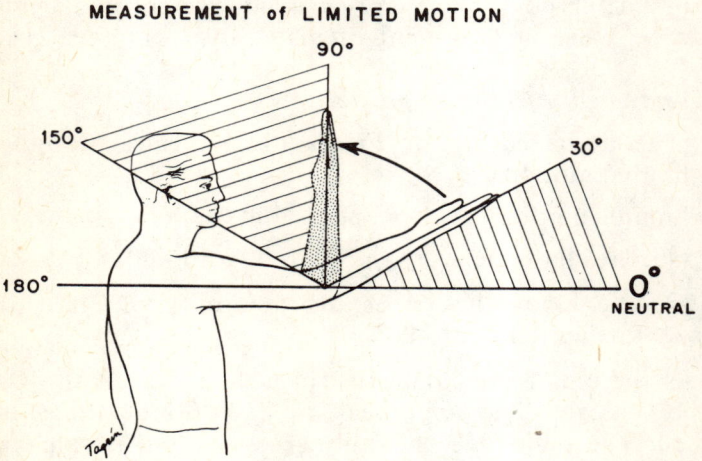

Fig. 111   Elbow motion

148

Zero Starting Position: This is the vertical upright position, or "thumbs up" position, with the forearm at the side of the body, and the elbow flexed 90°.

PRONATION and SUPINATION

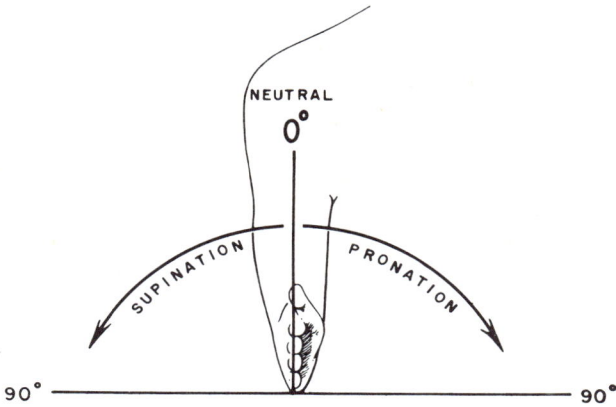

MEASUREMENT of LIMITED MOTION

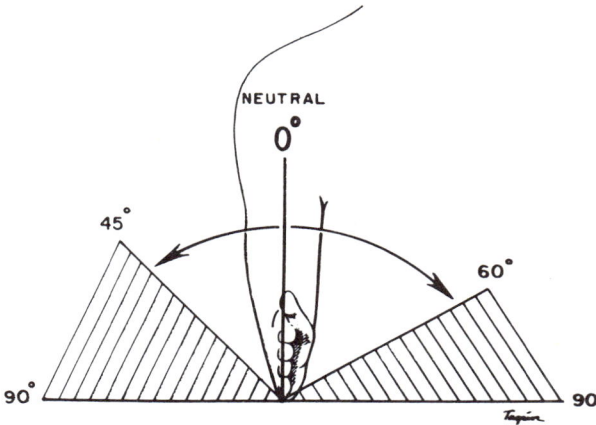

Fig. 112   Pronation and Supination

149

Pronation and Supination
Pronation = zero to 80°-90°
Supination = zero to 80°-90°
Total forearm motion = 160°-180°

Individuals may vary in the range of supination and pronation. Some individuals may reach the 90° arc, whereas others may have only 70° plus.

Limited Motion
Limited motion is simply expressed
Supination=45° (0°-45°)
Pronation=60° (0°-60°)
Total joint motion = 105°

Repeated and strained use of the wrist extensor muscles of the forearm may result in irritation of their origins at the lateral humeral condyle and this injury has commonly been designated by the term "*tennis elbow*." In addition to the tenderness noted at the muscular attachments to the lateral condyle, efforts to extend the wrist against resistance will result in pain in the muscles themselves and at their condylar attachments.

Injuries to both bones of the forearm, fractures and dislocations about the elbow, and the treatment applied for these injuries may result in compressive occlusion of the brachial artery or its branches in the forearm. Such occlusion if unrelieved for two or three hours will result in necrosis of the muscular and neural parts involved. The severity of the necrosis depends on the extent of the vascular occlusion, and *Volkmann's ischemic contracture* may occur. The signs of this impending disaster are the four "Ps."

1. Loss of the arterial *pulse* at the wrist.

2. *Pain* in the forearm and hand—accentuated by passive extension of the fingers.

3. *Pallor* of the fingers.

150

4. *Paralysis* as evidenced by inability to move the fingers.

Examination of such an extremity some days or weeks after this unrelieved complication has occurred will reveal contracture of the muscle-tendon units with resultant clawing of the fingers, flexion contracture of the wrist and impairment of nerve function of varying degree.

9. Wrist and Hand

The wrist joint is commonly defined as extending from a line one inch proximal to the articular surface of the radius distally to the carpometacarpal joints. Included are the radio-carpal joint, the distal radioulnar joint and the intercarpal joints. The joint surfaces provide maximal mobility and have no anatomical configuration to promote stability. That is provided entirely by the soft tissue structures, the collateral ligaments, articular disc, and interosseous ligaments. In spite of this, dislocation is not common and the result of injury to these joints is usually a fracture of one of several of the bone elements. Sprain or rupture of the ligaments is quite rare.

The bony landmarks are the radial styloid and the ulnar styloid with this latter the more proximal of the two. A line drawn between the two styloid processes lies at an angle of 15° with a line drawn perpendicular to the axis of the forearm. This relationship is disturbed in the frequently seen fracture of the distal radius *(Colles' fracture)* which when accompanied with the usually associated deformities of displacement and tilting of the distal radial fragment dorsally gives the familiar *silver fork deformity*.

The opposite deformity in a fracture in this same location is seen less commonly. Another fracture of the wrist, seen more commonly in the young adult, is fracture of the car-

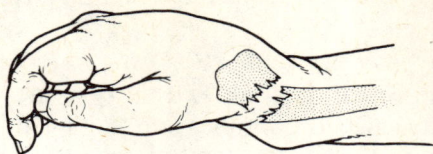

Fig. 113   Silver fork deformity—Colles Fracture

pal navicular and is demonstrated clinically by moderate swelling of the wrist and sharply localized tenderness over the navicular bone just distal to the radial styloid (anatomical *snuffbox*).

Dislocation may occur. The most common type is dislocation of the carpus dorsally with relation to the lunate which maintains its normal relationship to the radius. The dorsal displacement is noted by inspection and palpation and the normal relationship of the two styloid processes is not disturbed.

Motions

Zero Starting Position: The hand is in line with the forearm.

The natural motions of the wrist are flexion, extension, and ulnar and radial deviation from the zero starting position. Rotatory circumduction at the wrist occurs but can not be accurately measured.

Flexion: (palmar flexion) = 0°-80° ±
Extension: (dorsiflexion) = 0°-70° ±
Radial and Ulnar Deviation:
Radial Deviation = 0°-20°
Ulnar Deviation = 0°-30°

Ulnar deviation is usually measured with the wrist in pronation. When measured in supination, there is some increase in ulnar deviation.

FLEXION and EXTENSION

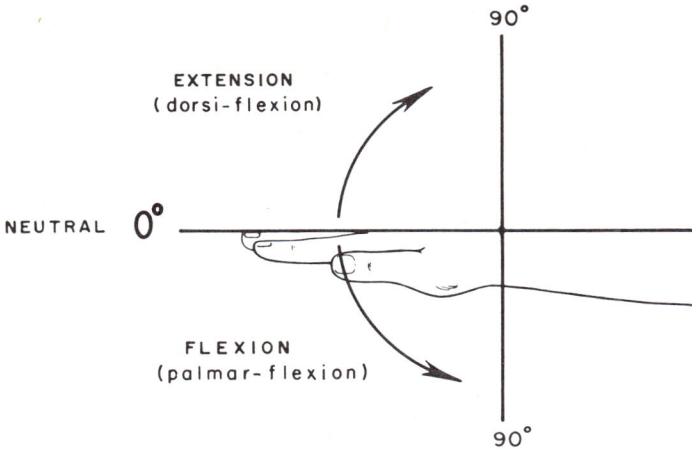

EXTENSION
(dorsi-flexion)

NEUTRAL 0°

FLEXION
(palmar-flexion)

90°

90°

RADIAL and ULNAR DEVIATION

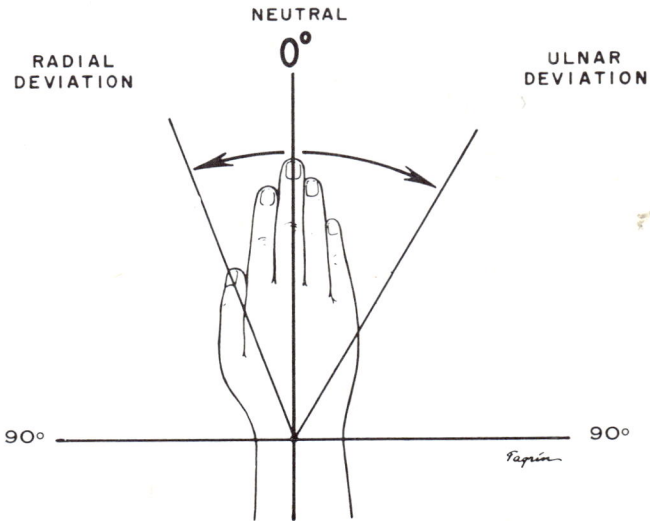

NEUTRAL
0°

RADIAL
DEVIATION

ULNAR
DEVIATION

90°

90°

Fig. 114   Wrist motions

153

Intra-articular fluid resulting from any articular inflammatory process may be demonstrated by swelling, the presence of tenderness especially noted dorsally, and restriction of wrist motion.

The tendons of the extensor pollicis brevis and the abductor pollicis longus cross the radial styloid in a common sheath and at times may be mechanically irritated by repetitive movements of the thumb so that the sheath becomes inflamed and swollen, compressing the two tendons (*DeQuervain's Disease*). The swelling is usually visible and is quite tender over a sharply localized area. Movement of the tendons may be associated with crepitus.

On the volar side of the wrist, the median nerve may be compressed beneath the transverse carpal ligament in the carpal canal. This condition (*carpal tunnel syndrome*) is seen most commonly in women in the fifth and sixth decades with the complaints usually being pain, numbness and weakness in the distribution of the median nerve. Hyper- or hyp-esthesia is usually demonstrable. Sharp percussion of the nerve in the canal may result in a tingling sensation along the distribution of the nerve in the hand. Atrophy of the thenar muscles may occasionally be demonstrated.

As the bones of the hand are subcutaneous, any fracture with displacement of the fragments is easily noted and is accompanied by the other signs of fracture. Similarly dislocations are noted by inspection and palpation.

Rupture or laceration of the tendons of the hand is common and is demonstrated by failure of the involved unit to move its skeletal insertion when the muscle portion contracts actively. At times, the ends of the ruptured tendon may be palpable. Rupture or laceration of a tendon of the flexor digitorum superfiscialis may be concealed through the ability of the flexor profundus to flex both distal and proximal interphalangeal joints. Isolation of profundus and superfiscialis function may be demonstrated by grasping and maintaining all of the digits except the one to be tested in strong extension. An attempt is then made to flex the digit being tested. With an intact superfiscialis, the digit will flex actively at the proximal interphalangeal joint but not at the distal interphalangeal joint. If the superfiscialis tendon is not intact, any attempt to actively flex the digit will not produce flexion.

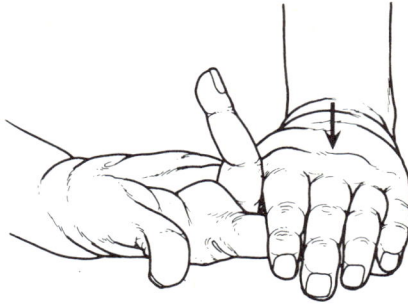

Fig. 115   Testing of flexor sublimus function

Avulsion of the attachment of the extensor tendon of one of the fingers frequently results from a sudden blow on the tip of the extended finger *(baseball finger, mallet finger)* and like any tendon rupture may be demonstrated by loss of function and the added evidence of hemorrhage and swelling resulting from the fracture.

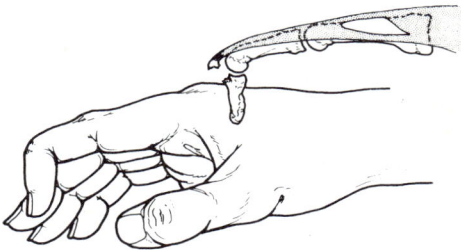

Fig. 116   Mallet finger

Thickening with later contracture of the slips of the palmar fascia is indicative of *Dupuytren's contracture.* Involvement is usually limited to the ring or little finger or both.

155

Boutonniere deformity results from a rupture of the central tendinous slip of the extensor hood with some tearing of the oblique fibers so that the lateral bands slip volarward, anterior to the axis of rotation of the PIP joint.

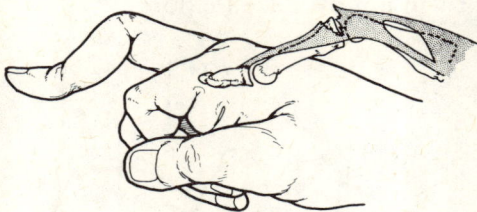

Fig. 117   Boutonniere deformity

Swan-neck deformity of the finger is the result usually of rheumatoid arthritis with contracture of the intrinsic muscles of the hand. The **MP** joint is fixed in flexion, the **PIP** joint is fixed in hyperextension and the **DIP** is in flexion because of extensor rupture or laxity.

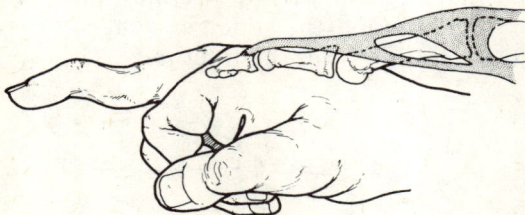

Fig. 118   Swan-neck deformity

Clawing of the fingers is the result of the loss of intrinsic muscle function usually from impaired medial and ulnar nerve function. The overaction of the extrinsic muscles takes the digit into hyperextension at the MP joint and into flexion at the PIP and DIP joints.

156

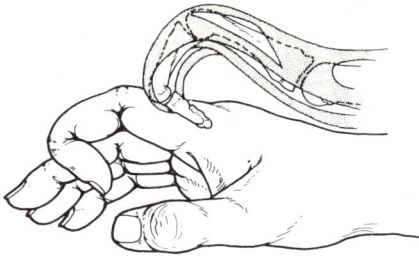

Fig. 119 Claw finger deformity

Trigger finger, seen most frequently in the ring finger, develops as the result of low grade inflammation of the proximal fold of the flexor tendon sheath, usually mechanical in origin. The tendon sheath thickens and causes at the same time local nodular swelling in the tendon. As a result, a triggering mechanism is set up so that the nodular swelling of the tendon is resisted as it attempts to pass through the thickened constricted portion of the sheath. Each excursion causes a distinct snap and at times the finger may finally be locked either in flexion or in extension. In addition to the typical snapping action, palpation at the base of the finger will disclose a nodule and the sensation of snapping is felt as the finger is flexed and extended.

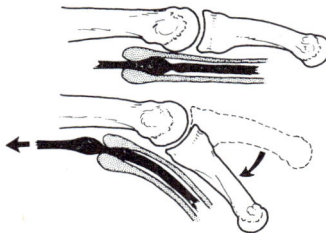

Fig. 120 Mechanism of trigger finger

Because of the multiple digits and joints in the hand and the importance of noting any changes in the mobility of the parts, motion, both active and passive, is carefully measured and promptly recorded.

10. Fingers

Nomenclature

In order to avoid mistaken identity, the fingers and thumb are referred to by name, rather than by number. Anatomical nomenclature is used for joints of the fingers and thumbs. Some surgeons prefer to use simpler terms for the fingers (noted in parenthesis).

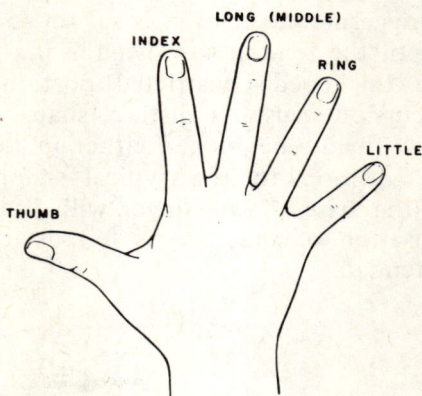

THE HAND

Fig. 121A
NOMENCLATURE
of FINGERS

Joints of the Fingers

a. The distal interphalangeal joint, the DIP joint (the distal joint).
b. The proximal interphalangeal joint, the PIP joint, (the middle joint).
c. Metacarpophalangeal joint, the MP joint, (the proximal joint).

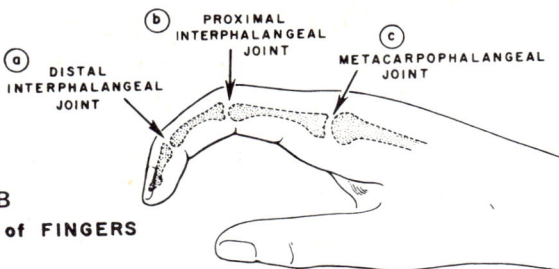

Fig. 121B
JOINTS of FINGERS

a. DISTAL INTERPHALANGEAL JOINT
b. PROXIMAL INTERPHALANGEAL JOINT
c. METACARPOPHALANGEAL JOINT

Joints of the Thumb
  a. Interphalangeal joint.
  b. Metacarpophalangeal joint.
  c. Carpometacarpal joint.

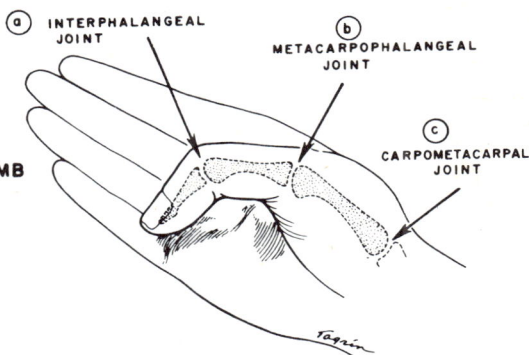

Fig. 121C
JOINTS of THUMB

a. INTERPHALANGEAL JOINT
b. METACARPOPHALANGEAL JOINT
c. CARPOMETACARPAL JOINT

Thumb
Motions: The motions of the thumb are complex and all definitions are necessarily somewhat arbitrary. The principal motions are: adduction, flexion, extension and opposition (circumduction).

Abduction and Adduction:

Zero Starting Position: The thumb is extended along the side of the index finger, which is in line with radius. (Fig. 122).

159

Abduction is defined as the angle created between the metacarpal bones of the thumb and the index finger. This motion may take place in two planes.

A—Illustrates zero starting position.

B—Illustrates abduction away from the plane of the palm with the hand in supination; the thumb points to the ceiling.

C—Illustrates abduction parallel to the plan of the palm (abduction-extension).

ZERO STARTING POSITION

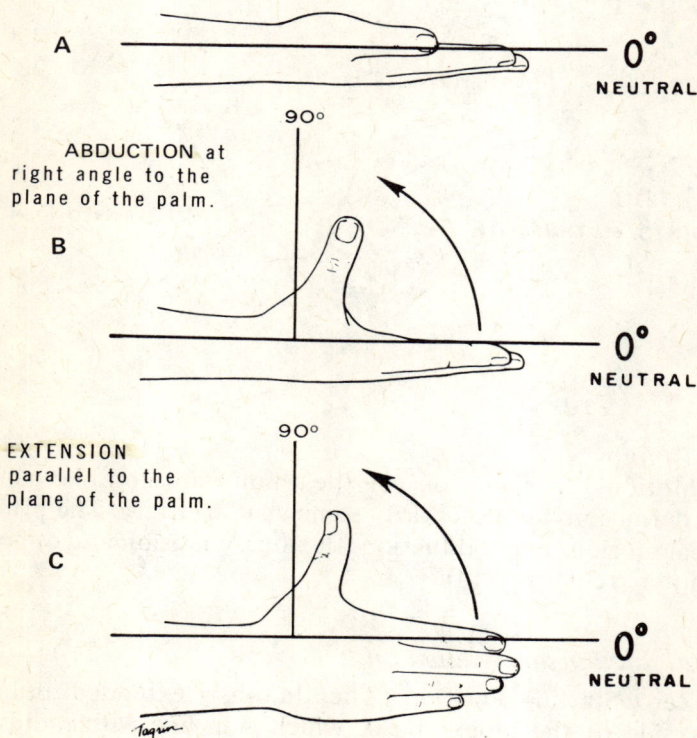

Fig. 122   Motions of the thumb

160

Flexion and Extension:

Zero Starting Position: The extended thumb.
Flexion of the interphalangeal joint:
    0°-80°

Flexion of Metacarpophalangeal joint:
    0°-50°
Flexion of carpometacarpal joint:
    0°-15°

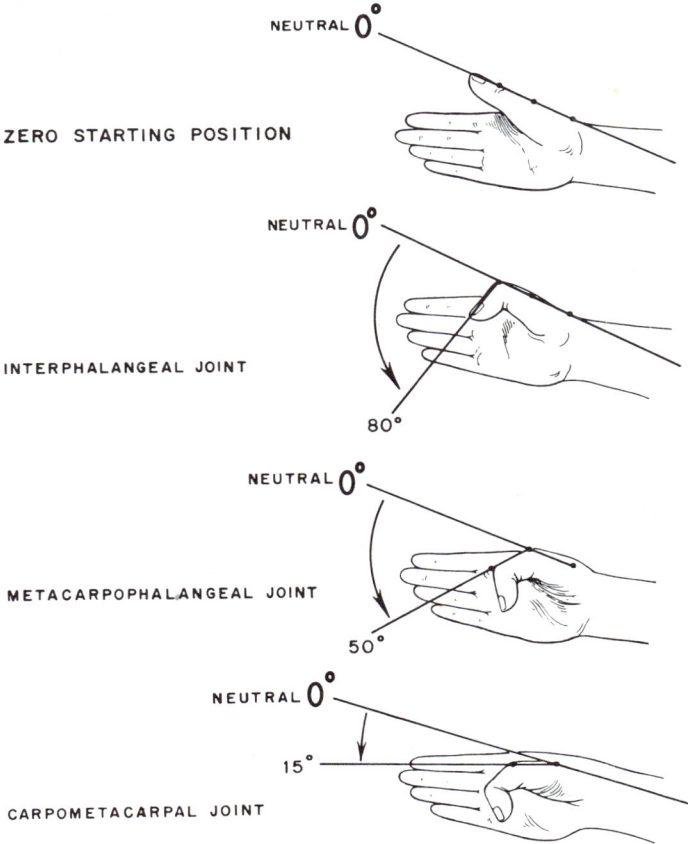

Fig. 123   Flexion of the thumb

Opposition

Zero starting postion: The extended thumb in line with the index fingers.

Opposition is a composite motion consisting of three elements:

(1) Abduction
(2) Rotation
(3) Flexion

This motion is usually considered complete when the tip, or pulp, of the thumb touches the tip of the fifth finger. Some surgeons, however, consider the arc of opposition complete when the tip of the thumb touches the base of the fifth finger. Both methods are illustrated.

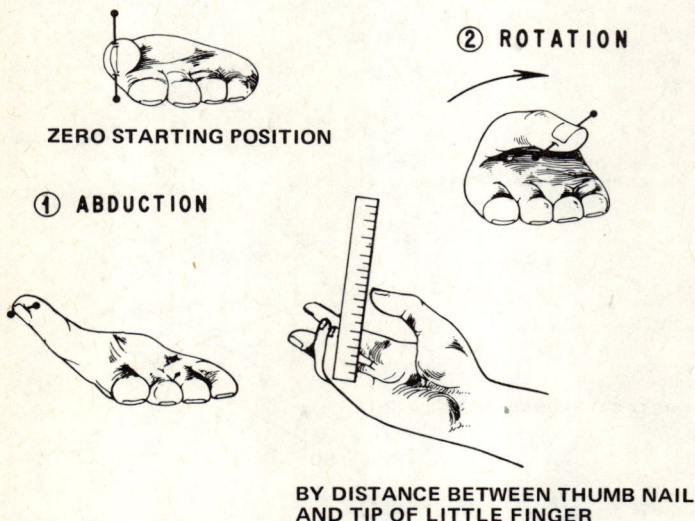

ZERO STARTING POSITION

① ABDUCTION

② ROTATION

BY DISTANCE BETWEEN THUMB NAIL
AND TIP OF LITTLE FINGER

Fig. 124A Opposition of the thumb and its measurement

Measurement of Opposition

This can be measured in centimeters or inches, from the tip of the thumb to the tip of the fifth finger or from the tip of the thumb, to the base of the fifth finger.

162

③ and FLEXION

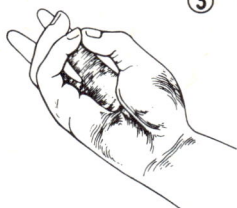

FLEXION TO TIP OF
LITTLE FINGER

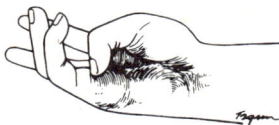

OR

FLEXION TO BASE OF
LITTLE FINGER

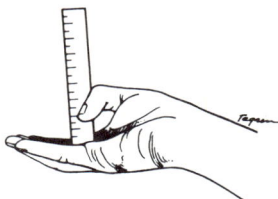

BY DISTANCE BETWEEN THUMB
AND BASE OF LITTLE FINGER

Fig. 124B Opposition of the thumb and its measurement

Flexion

Zero Starting Position: The extended fingers parallel to each other, and in line with the plane of the dorsum of the hand and wrist.

This motion can be estimated in degrees or in centimeters. Flexion is a natural motion in all joints of the fingers.

Composite motion of flexion.

This motion can be measured by a ruler, as the distance from the tip of the finger (indicate: (1) midpoint of pad or (2) nail edge) to the:

a. distal palmar crease (this measures flexion of the middle and distal joints).

b. proximal palmar crease (this measures flexion of the distal, middle and proximal joints of the fingers).

Fig. A

DISTAL INTERPHALANGEAL JOINT

90°

0°
NEUTRAL

0°
NEUTRAL

PROXIMAL INTERPHALANGEAL JOINT

100°

0°
NEUTRAL

METACARPOPHALANGEAL
JOINT

90°

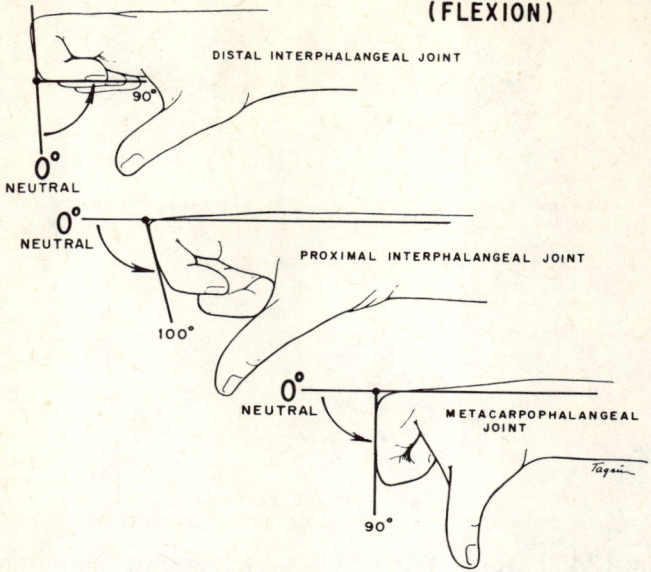

Fig. B COMPOSITE MOTION of FLEXION

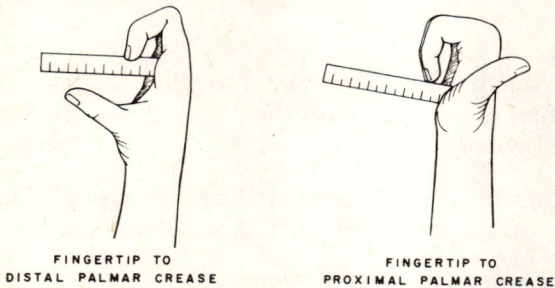

FINGERTIP TO
DISTAL PALMAR CREASE

FINGERTIP TO
PROXIMAL PALMAR CREASE

Fig. 125 Finger flexion and measurement

Extension

Extension with or without hyperextension is a natural
motion at the metacarpophalangeal joint, but not at the
proximal or distal interphalangeal joints.

164

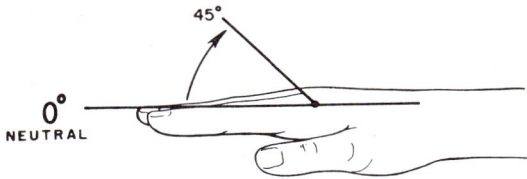

EXTENSION – METACARPOPHALANGEAL JOINT

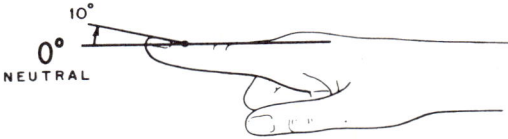

HYPEREXTENSION – DISTAL INTERPHALANGEAL JOINT

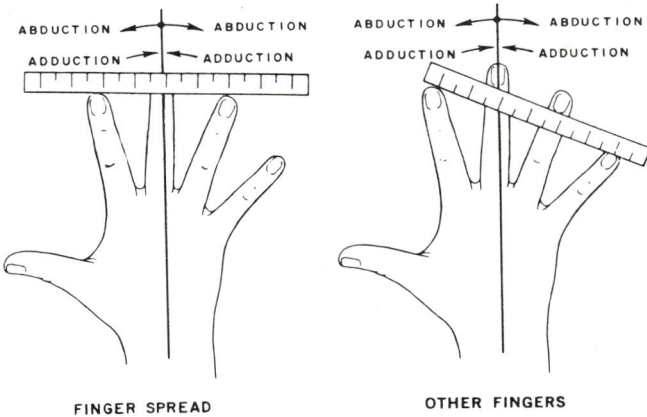

FINGER SPREAD

OTHER FINGERS

Fig. 126   Finger extension, abduction-adduction

Abduction and Adduction

(Finger Spread). This motion takes place in the plane of the palm away from and to the long or middle finger of the hand. It can be indicated in centimeters or inches, and measured between the tips of the little and index fingers or between the tips of other indicated fingers.

165

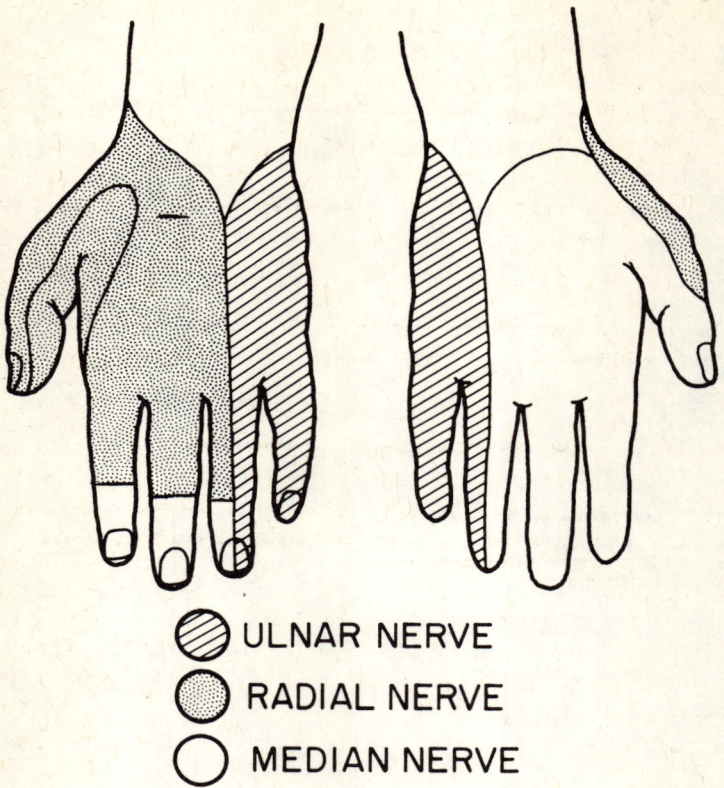

ULNAR NERVE

RADIAL NERVE

MEDIAN NERVE

Fig. 127   Sensory map of the hand

INITIAL CARE OF THE MULTIPLE INJURY PATIENT

In our mechanized society of today, severe and multiple injuries of the skeleton are seen frequently in combination with severe injuries of the other body systems. The emergency ward physician must be prepared to rapidly assess these injuries and at the same time initiate treatment procedures if the patient is to survive. Although multiple fractures of the extremities may be the most obvious injuries, they are frequently not immediately life-threatening, and they may be momentarily disregarded to check in regular, but in rapid fashion the other body systems that may present with injuries that immediately threaten life. These systems are checked in order of their importance:

1. Respiratory System

Respiratory failure is the most common cause of early death after injury so the first requirement is to check the respiratory system:

a. *Apnea:* If the patient is not breathing, mouth-to-mouth resuscitation should be initiated until a respirator is available or the patient breathes on his own. Oxygen should be delivered initially by mask, and then subsequently through an endotracheal tube.

b. *Obstruction:* If respiratory movement of the chest is seen but not effective, it is likely because of airway obstruction. This may be due to aspirated food particles, the tongue, blood, etc. A quick search should be made for these objects and their removal accomplished. An endotracheal tube is passed as soon as possible. Under hospital conditions, an emergency tracheotomy is rarely required.

c. *Ineffective Respiration:* As soon as a patient's airway is verified, if respiration is still ineffective, a search should be made for the following causes of difficulty:

(1) Open sucking wound — should be closed by a sterile dressing immediately.

167

(2) *Tension pneumothorax*—as evidenced by an expanded hemithorax and mediastinal shift. Emergency relief is obtained by needle aspiration and should be followed by sealed tube insertion.

(3) *Hemothorax and hemopneumothorax*—may vary from a small laceration of pulmonary parenchyma that will heal spontaneously to major vessel laceration or rupture. If paradoxical respiration is evident as the cause of ineffective respiration, it requires emergency aspiration and tube insertion.

(4) *Flail chest*—use of a positive pressure respirator via endotracheal tube is urgent

2. Circulatory System

With an adequate airway established, the heart beat should be checked by palpation, by ausculation, and as soon as possible, by electrocardiograph monitor. If it is not beating, external cardiac massage is instituted and continued rhythmically until restoration of an effective heart beat.

By far the most common cause of acute circulatory failure is hemodynamic *shock*. Acute shock is the result of blood loss. When present, it indicates a loss in excess of one-quarter of the blood volume. This loss should be replaced while its cause is found and arrested.

a. *External Bleeding:* This bleeding may be controlled temporarily by pressure.

At the same time a vein is entered either by needle or openly by cannula, blood is drawn for typing and cross match, and immediately an infusion of saline, lactated Ringer's, or plasma is pumped in rapidly until the blood pressure is restored. As soon as matched blood is available, it is given in addition to the initial fluids until a normal blood volume is restored. As soon as replacement is underway, a search is made for sources of internal bleeding.

b. *Internal Bleeding:*

(1) Thorax: There are usually external signs of blunt trauma, expansion of the involved side of the chest, and accompanying signs of respiratory distress. Immediate needle aspiration and insertion of a sealed tube are done. If subsequent examination shows that bleeding in the thorax alone has produced the shock, then a major vessel injury has occurred and surgical repair should be considered. A common cause is rupture of the thoracic aorta by steering wheel impact.

(2) Abdomen: Intra-abdominal bleeding is shown early by muscle spasm and absent bowel sounds. Quadrant taps for evidence of blood should follow. Evidence of free blood in the peritoneal cavity demands emergency exploration.

(3) Urinary Tract: Bleeding from the urinary tract is rarely an emergency and alone is not likely to be the cause of shock. However, genito-urinary bleeding frequently indicates severe associated closed pelvic fractures. Fractures of this vascular cancellous bone can rapidly fill the pelvis with 25-50% of the blood volume. Bladder catheterization should be done immediately and pelvic fractures sought as soon as the acute examination is finished.

(4) Central Nervous System: Bleeding here is usually not of itself the cause of shock. Other systems that are the source of bleeding should not be overlooked. In skull fracture, emergency craniotomy to control and relieve epidural hemorrhage may sometimes be required, but not to control acute circulatory collapse from shock.

(5) Extremities: Concealed hemorrhage from multiple major fractures is a common cause of acute shock. The adult thigh may contain 25% of the blood volume thirty minutes after a fracture of the femur. A conservative estimate is 1000 cc per major fracture. Continuous bleeding can be determined by serial circumferential measurements. Pulselessness of an extremity means arteriography should be considered if realignment and stabilization of fractures do not afford relief.

169

c. *Response to Treatment:* The acute shock status is best monitored by:

    (1) Blood pressure and pulse,
    (2) Central venous pressure, and
    (3) Measurement of urinary output every hour by catheter.

Only after there has been adequate response to this emergency review and treatment, is time utilized to evaluate the patient system-by-system in a more thorough manner for evidence of less urgent although equally severe injuries. This more detailed examination includes viewing and palpating all body surfaces, if this has not already been done.

1. Thorax. A chest x-ray is made to confirm and deliniate life-threatening injuries. Their acute care has already been discussed. Suction via the endotracheal tube should be repeated gently to maintain the airway.

2. Abdomen. The most frequent injuries are ruptures of the spleen, liver, or intestines. Bleeding from one of these organs may not produce symptoms for some time and may be responsible for lack of response to shock treatment.

3. Head and Central Nervous System. Since acute surgery is only required for:

    (a) Expanding hematomas,
    (b) An open skull fracture, or
    (c) A depressed skull fracture; head-injured patients need a baseline evaluation early so that improvement or deterioration can be quickly noted. This baseline includes:

        1) Level of consciousness.
        2) Localized neurological deficits such as:
            a. Cranial nerve involvement including pupillary response and ocular movements, and
            b. Paresis or hemiparesis.

The patient is closely watched for evidence of increasing intracranial pressure manifested by:

(1) Slowing pulse and respiration, and

(2) Blood pressure elevation.

Skull films, computerized tomography, and arterior-grams may be done for complete study when the patient is otherwise stabilized.

3. **Genito-Urinary System.** The diagnosis of injury of the genito-urinary system depends upon the demonstration of bloody urine, either gross or microscopic. Radiographic studies may be required to locate the origin. Early operative intervention is indicated for bladder rupture.

4. **Spine and Extremities.** Patients who have had skull injuries or complain of neck pain should be considered as potentially having a cervical spine injury. They should be protected (traction, manual or mechanical) until definitive x-rays are available. Patients with back signs or symptoms should be regarded as potentially having a spine fracture until adequate x-rays are seen.

Unless the neurological examination indicates cord injury, vertebral fractures and dislocations do not require emergency reduction. They do require careful protection while moving the patient to determine the extent of neurologic involvement and to obtain x-rays.

For the extremities, emergency management demands:

a. Control of bleeding by external pressure,

b. Restoration of impaired circulation by traction or manipulation,

c. Preparation for the control of threatened infection from open wounds by the use of masks and gloves during examination and early coverage with sterile dressings, and

d. Proper splinting of fractures. Distressingly, the subsequent treatment of fractures is often made more difficult by their displacement after arrival at the hospital. This is due to lack of proper splinting while other examinations, x-rays, transfer to treatment area, etc., are being

171

done. Splints should be applied to *all* suspected fractures until their presence is excluded or definitive treatment is accomplished. The most common is the plastic "air" splint, which is quickly inflated, and allows good x-ray interpretation with the splint in place.

Open fractures require debridement and dressing as soon as possible since the incidence of osteomyelitis increases with each hour of undebrided contamination.

Following this assessment of the patient, the priorities of his injuries are determined. Patients with multiple system injuries, like any other patient, must have a responsible attending physician. Too often these patients receive care from a "system" standpoint and their overall care suffers. The doctor who is responsible should be determined as soon as the acute examination and care are concluded. It then becomes the responsibility of the patient's physician to provide general care including tetanus immunization, antibiotic therapy, order of care, and postoperative management. While this is frequently a "team" effort, the team must have a clearly defined quarterback.

LABORATORY AIDS
IN ORTHOPAEDIC MANAGEMENT

Laboratory tests are most often used in the care of orthopaedic patients (1) to help diagnose the patient's disease, (2) to screen the functional capacity of other body systems prior to major surgery and (3) to monitor physiologic processes after surgery or injury.

The tests are not substitutes for a thorough history and physical examination. Their value depends upon the thought that goes into their selection and their interpretation in light of the clinical findings. The patient's physician may wish consultation from others with special competence, but as the final decision is his, knowledge of the value and limitation of laboratory tests is essential.

1. Diagnostic Examinations:

a. X-rays are the most common laboratory examination used to aid in the diagnosis of musculoskeletal conditions.

Roentgenographic examination of the involved or symptomatic part is nearly always indicated—frequently to either confirm or rule out clinical impressions. In addition, it is useful to search out asymptomatic involvement that is suspected clinically i.e., metastatic skeletal involvement, chest metastasis, patterns of metabolic disease in the sites of most common manifestation. X-rays, like all laboratory tests, should not be ordered as a routine but should be obtained for a definite reason.

The x-ray films in all likelihood will be reviewed by a radiologist for his consulting opinion. His consultation will be greatly enhanced by informing him of the specific purpose of obtaining the films. The physician responsible for the patient should personally view the films and interpret what he sees and in consultation with the radiologist decide if additional views or special studies are indicated.

Some of the more common special studies are:

(1) *Planograms (Laminograms)*: These are used to bring out fine details of a process that can be obscured by overlying radiopaque bone.

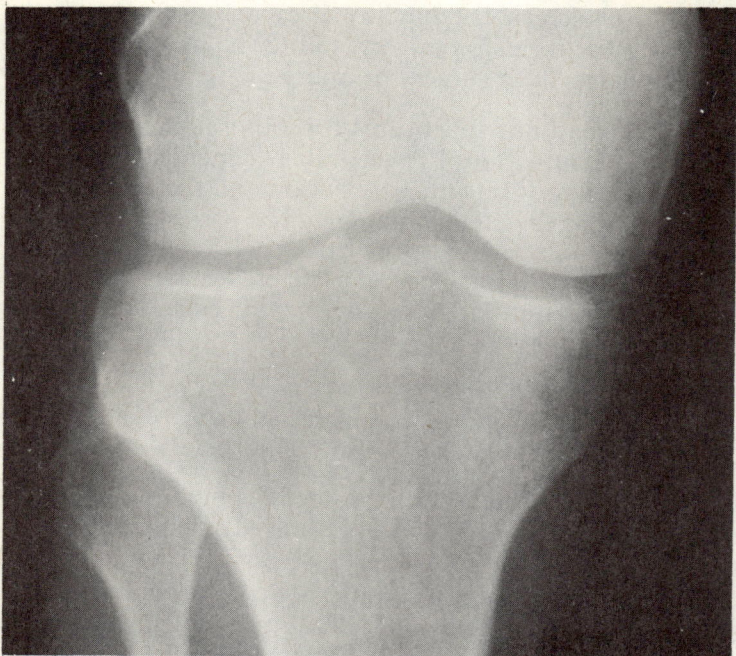

Fig. 128 A) A-P Tibia

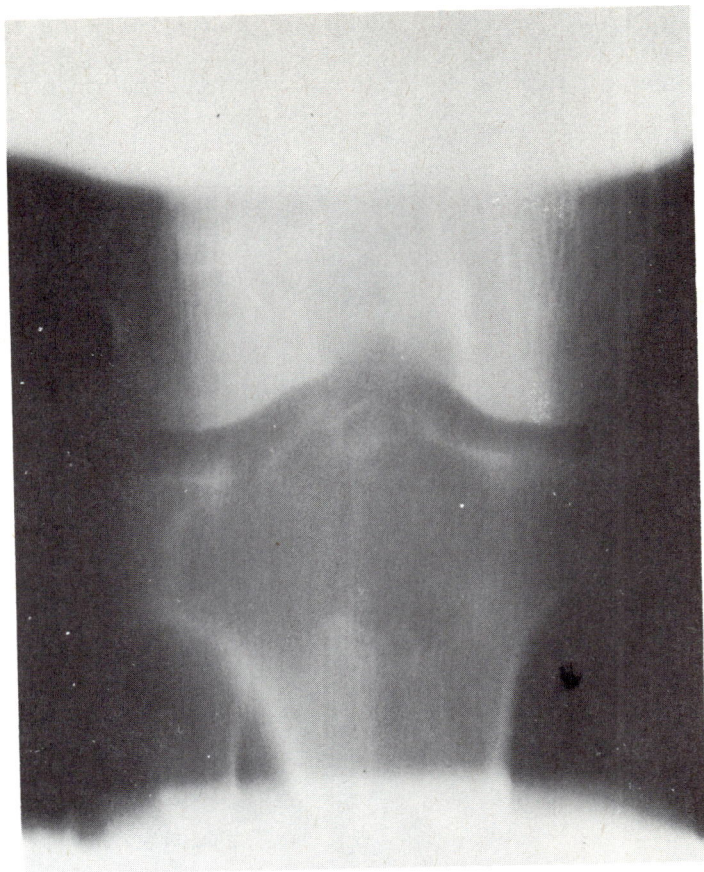

Fig. 128   B) Planogram

The details of a giant cell tumor
are brought by the planogram.

(2) *Myelograms:* These are x-rays following injection of inert radiopaque dyes or radiolucent gases to outline soft tissue defects along the spinal canal or in the skull.

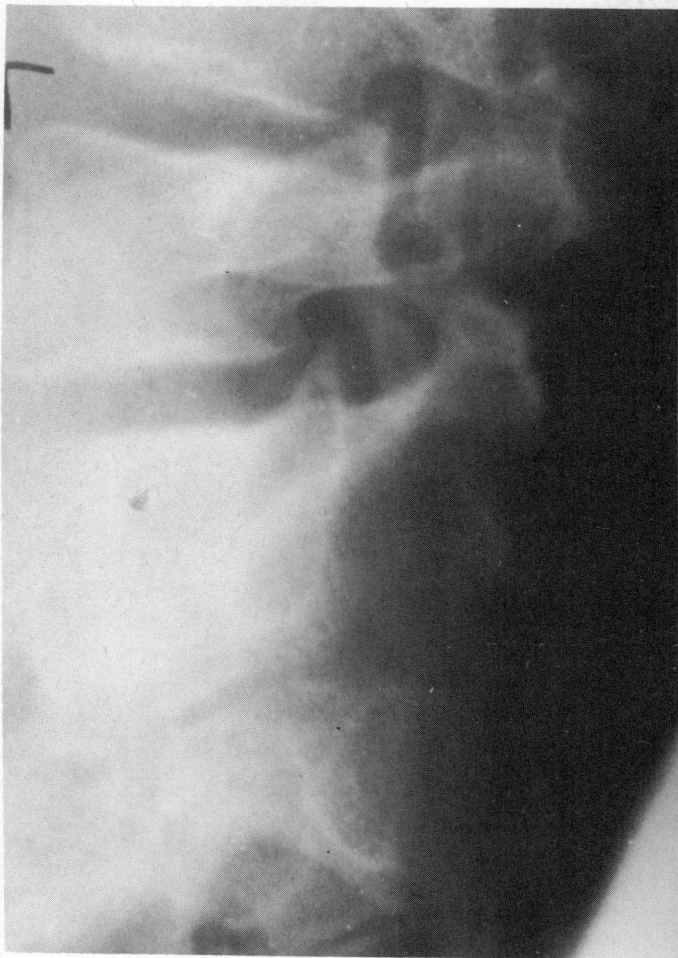

Fig. 129 A) Oblique Lumbar Spine

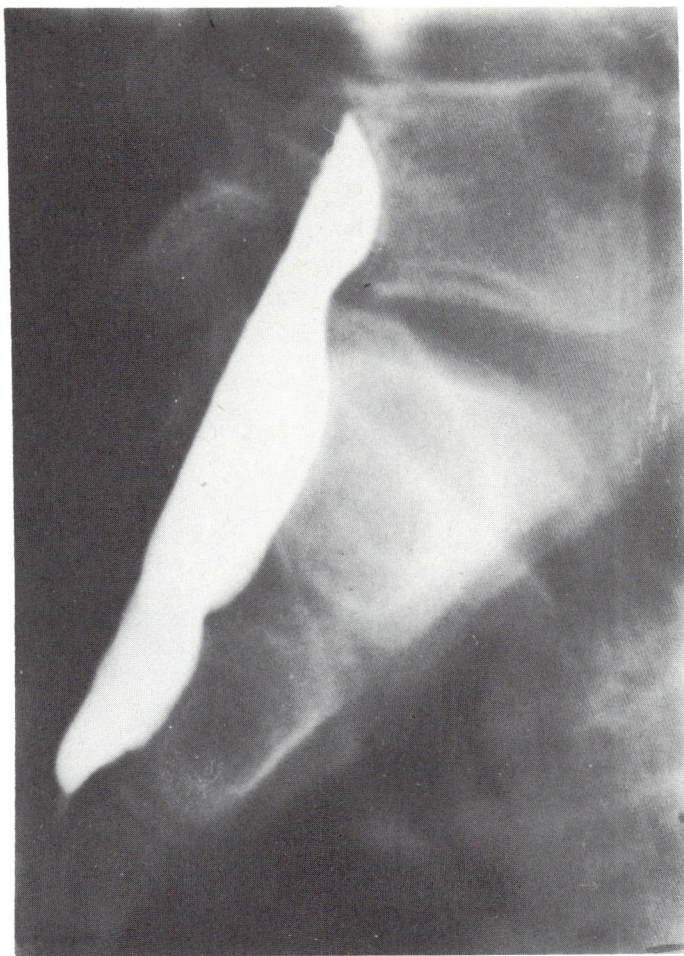

Fig. 129 B) Myelogram

The bulge in the dye column represents the
posterior aspect of the intervertebral disc.

(3) *Arthrograms:* These are x-rays made after injection of radiopaque dyes or radiolucent gases into joints to outline soft tissue defects or masses.

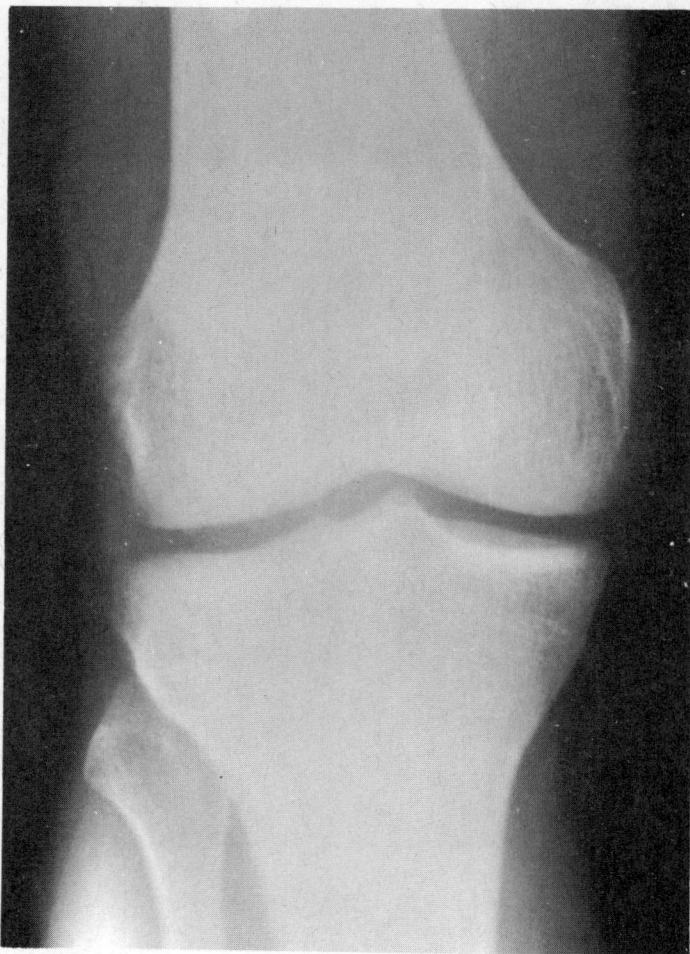

Fig. 130 A) A-P Knee

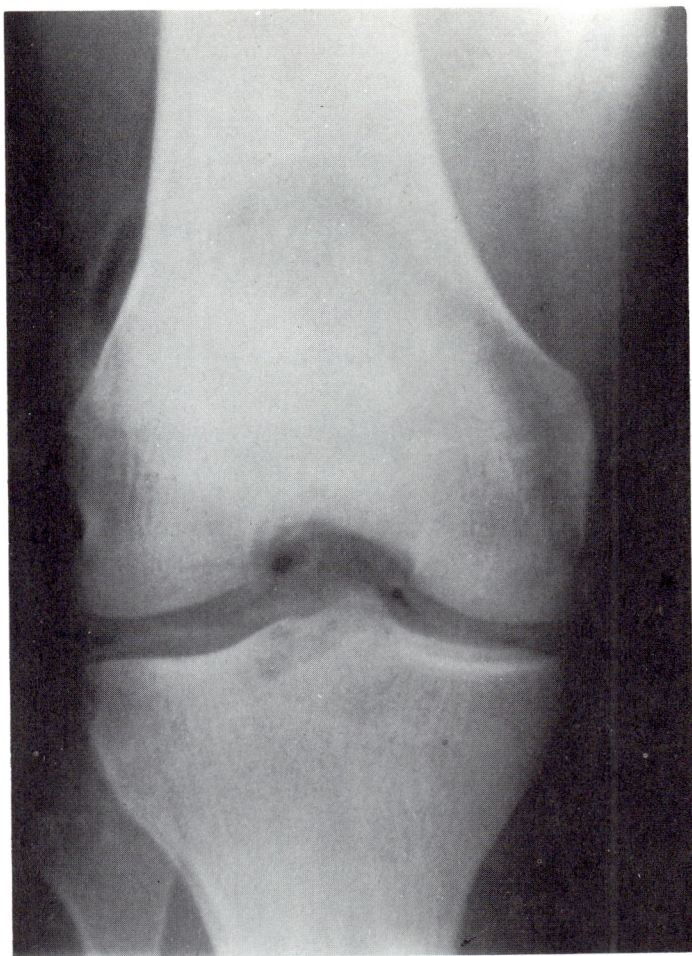

Fig. 130 B) Arthrogram

The air injected into the knee joint outlines the
radiolucent articular cartilages and menisci.

(4) *Sinograms:* X-rays made after injecting draining sinuses with radiopaque dyes may show where the draining sinuses go in the deeper tissues and what their ramifactions may be.

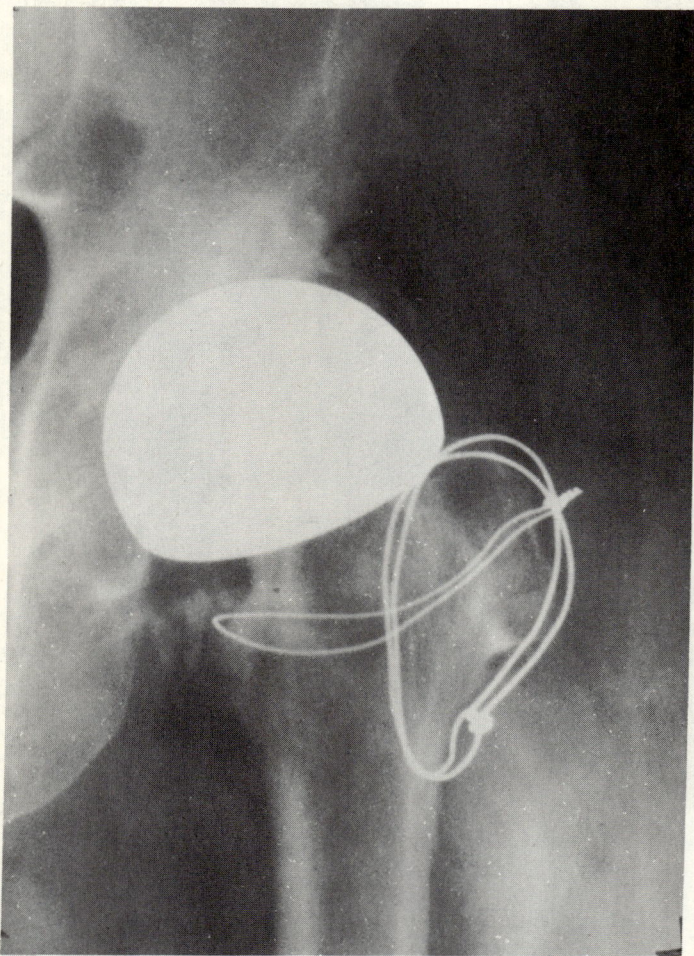

Fig. 131 A) A-P Hip

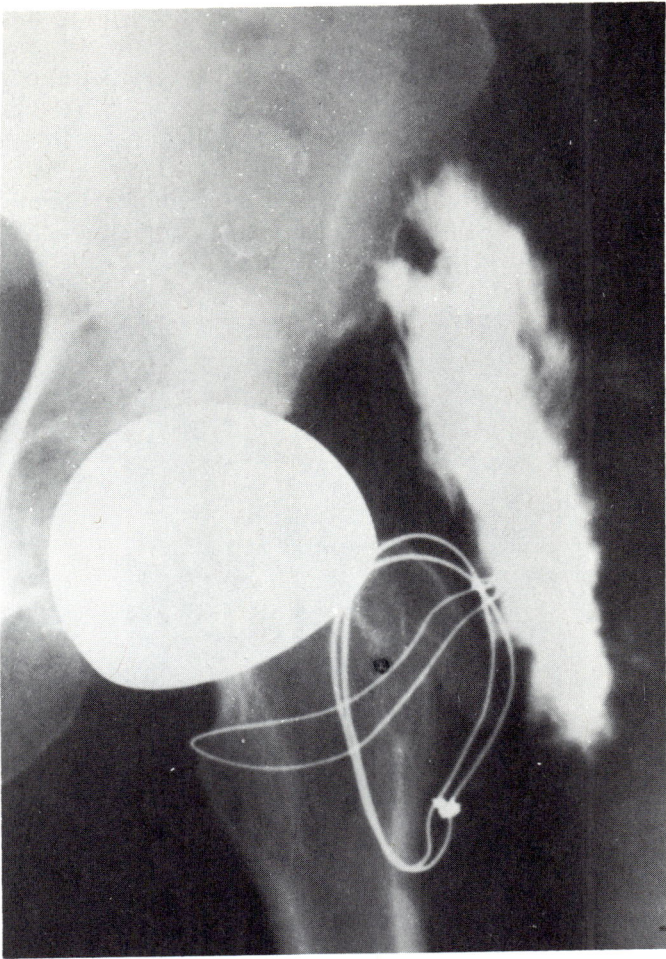

Fig. 131 B) Sinogram

Dye injected into a draining sinus
outlines the extent of a deep abscess.

(5) *Angiograms:* X-rays made after injecting major vessels with radio-opaque dyes demonstrate abnormal vascular patterns and are helpful in assessing post-traumatic vascular deficits and accurately localizing soft tissue neoplasms. With these and CAT and isotope scans, the surgeon may accurately construct a three-dimensional model of a tumor that greatly facilitates surgical planning. Venograms are also useful to supplement myelography in the diagnosis of nerve root syndromes.

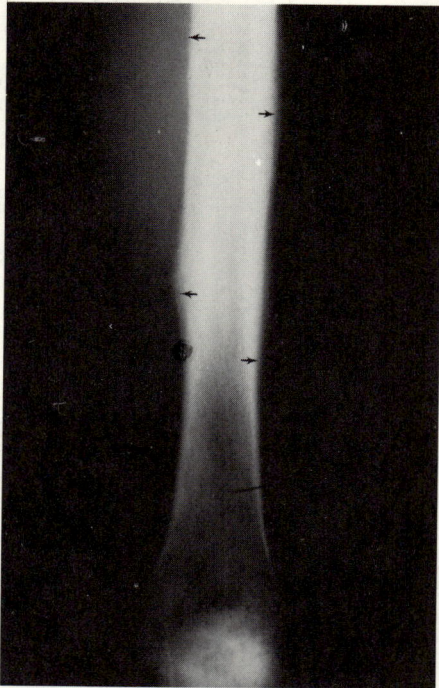

Fig. 132A

(A) A 20-year-old male with a Ewing's sarcoma of the femoral shaft. Arrows indicate involvement of the mid-third of the femur with modest periosteal reaction.

182

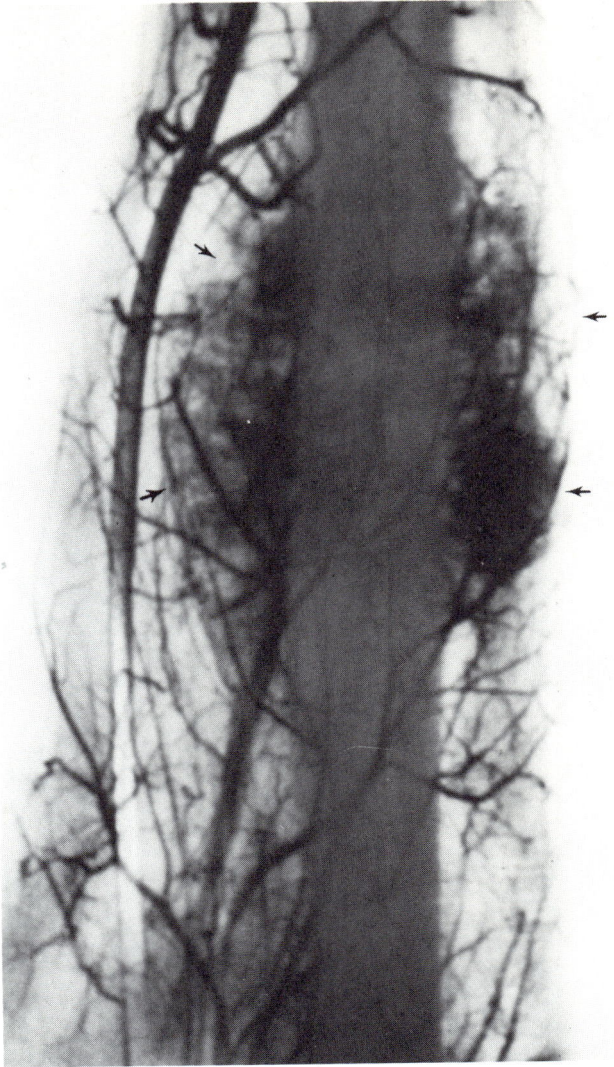

Fig. 132B

(B) Angiogram: Arrows indicate the extent of the soft tissue mass in the adjacent soft tissues.

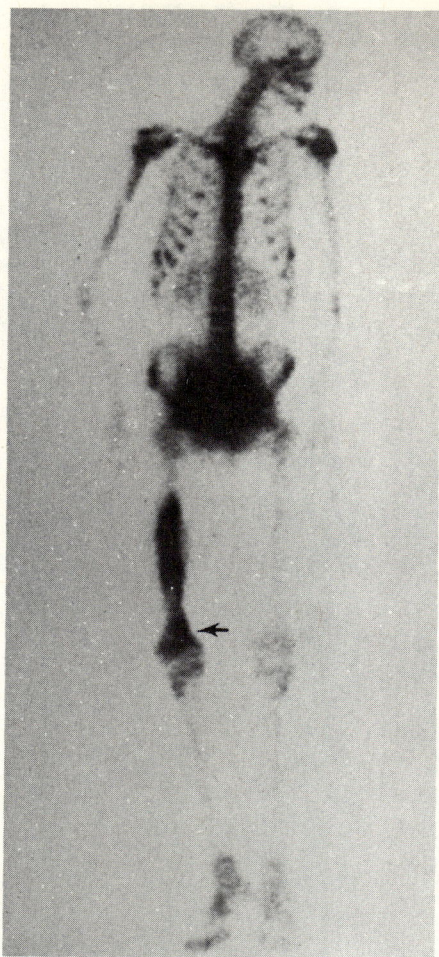

Fig. 133

This is a Tc_{99} scan of the patient whose X-ray and angiogram are shown in Figure 132. The mid-third of the femur seen to be involved by X-ray shows marked isotope uptake. A secondary area of involvement (arrow) in the distal femur, not seen on the X-ray, is shown on the scan.

184

(6) *Radioisotope Scanning:* Radiographic imaging of radioactive isotopes is widely used to detect areas of abnormal bone activity. The commonest isotope (technetium polyphosphate) used in bone scanning has a short duration (half-life of six hours) and a low body burden that permits repeated examination. The isotope uptake is increased by either an increase in blood supply (as it is an intravascular injection) or an increase in bone deposition (as the isotope is chelated at sites of mineralization). Its many uses are related to detecting alterations in bone blood supply (i.e. aseptic necrosis) or changes in bone activity. It is particularly useful in detecting small foci of intraosseous tumors in the face of normal X-rays. Rapid changes in technology are increasing both the accuracy and precision of radioisotope applications in this expanding field.

(7) *Computerized Axial Tomography (CAT):* This produces cross-sectional X-rays by computers that project an image of bone and soft tissues. This method, while still evolving technically, has opened a new horizon and greatly improved the accuracy of determining a lesion's location in difficult areas such as the spine, pelvis, and shoulder girdle. When combined with angiography and isotope scanning, it makes possible the construction of three dimensional models of mass lesions and their relationships to anatomic compartments. It is also very useful in visualizing alterations within radiologically occult areas such as the spinal canal, medullary canal of long bones, pelvis, etc.

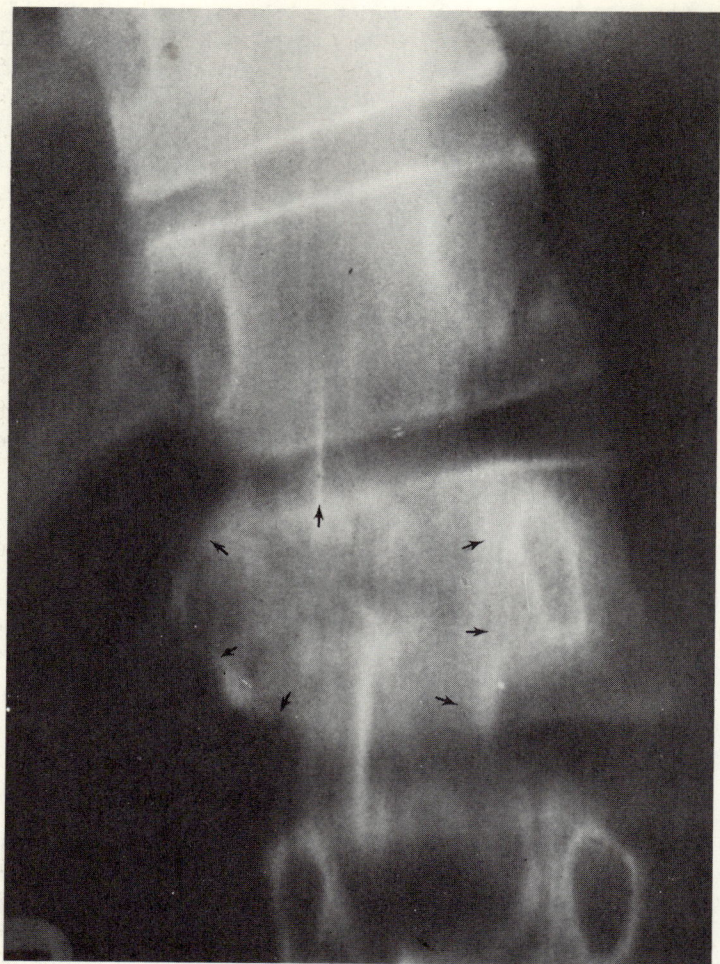

Fig. 134A

A 14-year-old girl with a painful scoliosis caused by a benign osteoblastoma of L_1.

Arrows indicate the involvement of the pedicle and body of the first lumbar vertebra.

186

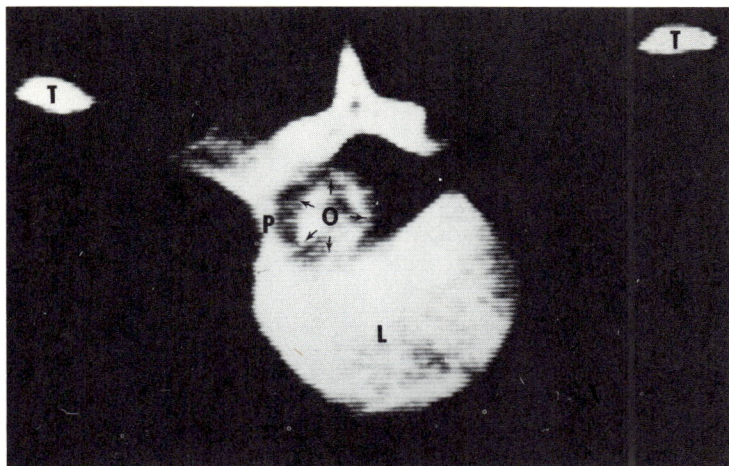

Fig. 134B

The extent of the lesion into the neural canal is clearly shown on the CAT scan. Such information is indispensable to accurate surgical planning.

(L = cross-section of the body of L_1; P = pedicles of L_1; T = transverse processes; O = extent of the osteoblastoma within the neural canal)

b. *Biopsies:* Histologic examination of tissues is frequently the focal point of diagnosis. Biopsies should be done for specific indications. The pathologist must be apprised of all the relevant clinical facts. The surgeon should personally view the tissues grossly and histologically to insure that representative material is available for examination. When the microscopic diagnosis is at great variance with the clinical suspicion, it is the surgeon's obligation to be certain that technical errors have not produced inadequate tissue for examination. In this regard frozen sections frequently help to ascertain the tissue adequacy and in many instances an accurate diagnosis. The surgeon further must be certain of the limitations of the histologic examination and not equate "consistent with" or "suggestive of" with "diagnostic of." This can only be done by close personal contact with the consulting pathologist.

c. *Arthroscopic Study:* The use of the arthroscope has given the orthopaedic surgeon the opportunity to study the internal structures of a joint without the potential morbidity that is attendant on a regular arthrotomy. The fine arthroscope may be inserted through a small skin stab wound and as the arthroscope is moved about from point to point any abnormalities in the joint may be noted. It has found its greatest usefulness in the study of the knee but it has been used in other joints of the body as well. As in other aspects of orthopaedic surgery the usefulness of arthroscopic examination will in great part be directly related to the experience and the skill of the surgeon employing this method of examination.

d. Biochemical Determinations: While routine screening of urine and blood samples is commonly done to exclude the possibility of common indicators such as leucocytosis, anemia, pyuria, overt diabetes, etc., these tests must be interpreted in light of the clinical situation. With the expansion of "multiphasic laboratory" screening tests, this clinical correlation will become increasingly important.

The clinical manifestations dictate which of the vast array of laboratory tests may be of significance in the diagnostic evaluation of a particular orthopaedic patient. However, because a large number of these patients present with problems that revolve around neurologic, muscle, bone, or synovial processes, discussion of the indications for and significance of certain studies is pertinent.

1. *Cerebro-spinal fluid:* Laboratory studies on cerebrospinal fluid are most often used to distinguish infections, neoplasms, and degenerative processes. The signifi-

cant findings are (1) increased cell counts and decreased amounts of glucose and chlorides in infections, (2) increased protein in tumors and (3) normal findings in degenerative processes such as multiple sclerosis. Syphilis, sought for because of Charcot joints, may be frequently confirmed by CSF in the presence of negative blood findings. Bloody spinal fluid indicates hemorrhage through the meninges (intracerebral or subarachnoid) in contrast to clear fluid under increased pressure associated with hemorrhage not rupturing the meninges (subdural hematoma). (Reference: Dandsohn, Israel: Henny, John B. (Editor), Todd-Sanford Clinical Diagnosis by Laboratory Methods. 19th Edition, 1969, W.B. Saunders Company.

2. *Synovial fluid:* As synovial fluid is normally a transudate of the serum, its analysis is most often used to distinguish inflammatory from degenerative types of arthritis. Since the synovial-cell membrane is intact in the degenerative processes, the findings reflect a transudate—high viscosity, few cells, good mucin clot, and elevated proteins. With rupture of the membrane by inflammatory lesions, the findings are those of an exudate—low viscosity, many cells, poor mucin clot, and decreased protein. Specific tests are urate crystals (gout), calcium pyrophosphate (pseudo-gout), cultures, and rheumatoid-like factors. (Reference: Cohen, Alan S. (Editor), Laboratory Diagnostic Procedures in the Rheumatic Diseases, 1967, Little, Brown and Company.)

3. *Muscle Enzymes:* Enzyme analysis is employed to distinguish muscle weakness due to dystrophic diseases of the muscle per se from the atrophic results of denervation. As indicated by the clinical picture, they are frequently combined with other special diagnostic tests as electromyography, nerve conduction studies, and muscle biopsy. In general, dystrophic lesions produce elevations in enzyme activity (aldolase and phosphocreatinkinase are the most commonly measured) while atrophic diseases show no increase in enzyme activity.

189

4. *Mineral Metabolism:* Of all the serum and urine examinations, the orthopaedic patient more commonly has levels of calcium, phosphorus, and alkaline phosphatase measured. While there are many other specific tests for various diseases of the musculoskeletal system that are of value, these tests are usually called for on specific grounds by the clinical picture to establish or deny a particular diagnosis.

Since *calcium and phosphorus* ion levels in the serum and urine are mirrors of skeletal metabolic activity, they are commonly used in differentiating diseases that cause altered skeletal density. Although the clinical and radiologic findings often indicate a gain or loss in skeletal mass, the ion levels may help distinguish the process that produces the abnormality. These levels are most commonly used when radiologically the bones lose density *(Osteopenia)* but the ionic pattern does not identify which of the many causes (osteoporosis, osteomalacia, renal disease, parathyroid hyperactivity, thyroid hyperactivity, rickets, myelomatosis, to mention only a few) is present.

Similarly, *alkaline phosphatase,* as an enzyme essential to mineralization of the organic bone matrix, reflects the amount of skeletal rebuilding activity—i.e., osteoblastic formation of new bone.

In order to obtain the most effective use of these tests, they must be used intelligently and not in a "shotgun" approach in reaction to an unexpected x-ray finding. Thus, a brief resume of their use and limitations is appropriate.

Calcium and phosphorus, both essential for basic life processes and the main mineral constituents of the skeleton, are transported in the blood and the determinations of their levels should be utilized in the diagnostic study of skeletal disease and injury.

Normal blood values:

Calcium: 8.5 - 10.5 mgm./100 ml. This consists of almost equal parts of ionizable and nonionizable protein-bound calcium. A small amount is combined with citric acid.

Phosphorus: 3 - 4.5 mgm./100 ml. This is the plasma phosphate, which is almost completely ionized in the plasma as H_2PO_4/HPO_4, one of the plasma buffer systems.

Calcium is obtained from foodstuffs, the most important of which is milk or milk products. The daily requirement is estimated at 600 mg. for the adult and is greater in the growing child, and in pregnancy and lactation. Calcium is absorbed from the small bowel, vitamin D being necessary for this absorption which is aided by bile. In addition to absorption, calcium is excreted into the bowel in the digestive juices, bile, pancreatic and salivary juices. With the average daily adult intake of 1,000 mg., about 800 to 900 mg. is excreted in the stools. However, rather than absorbing just 100 to 200 mg./day, the estimated 400 mg./day excreted in the digestive juices must be replaced so that 500 to 600 mg. is actually absorbed, although the net gain is still only 100 to 200 mg./day.

The mean adult urinary excretion of calcium is between 100 and 200 mg./day. Any values above 250 should be considered suspiciously, but these can only be categorized as high when the other factors of intake, bowel excretion, and metabolic regulation are considered. Only the calcium in the diffusable fraction passes the membrane of the glomerulus but more than 99% of this is reabsorbed in the tubules of the kidney.

Phosphorus is widely distributed in foodstuffs and intestinal absorption is more complete than that of calcium. Absorption is impaired by a high diet of calcium, by aluminum hydroxide and by beryllium. As plasma inorganic phosphate is completely ionized, all passes the glomerular filter. About 90% is absorbed in the proximal tubules. Both the plasma level and the daily excretion of phosphorus are more variable compared to calcium. These levels vary depending upon intake and the time of the day. With an ordinary intake, about 600 mg./day is excreted in the urine.

As 99% of the body calcium is found in the skeleton, a study of calcium balance, that is, the amount of calcium taken into the body in the food as related to the output in the feces and urine, indicates what is happening to calcium in the bone. Thus, this type of study can be used to determine whether calcium is being laid down, is being removed from bone, or is in balance in bone. This latter state does not mean that there is no calcium ion interchange in bone, but only that the amount taken up by bone is the same as the amount which is given up. Calcium and phosphorus are the important inorganic constituents of bone and exist in a crystalline form, *hydroxyapatite,* probably represented as $3 Ca_3(PO_4)_2 Ca(OH)_2$. The crystals are small, 40 Å x 250 Å x 60 Å, with some variance in size and with the unit cell of the lattice 9.4 x 9.4 x 6.9 Å. The small size and flat shape of the crystals give them a large surface area that allows for ready ionic interchange. The surface ions absorb ions from the body fluids which in turn bind a layer of water giving a hydration shell. Through the hydration shell enclosing the crystal, bone salt can take part in metabolic exchange. Ions within the crystal have a slower turnover rate than those of the surface. This constant ionic interchange is entirely in addition to the changes that take place with bone growth and remodeling.

5. *Bacteriologic Studies:* Smears and cultures for the identification of etiologic bacterial agents are essential in the diagnosis of septic processes. They must be used in the light of the clinical picture and with the knowledge of the normal flora of the region studied. The surgeon is obliged to provide the microbiologist with the same adequate material and information that he provides the pathologist. Prior consultation in methods of fixation, proper media and other factors rather than "routine smears, culture, and sensitivity" requests will frequently garner important information irrevocably missed by rote screening and inappropriate therapy. Sensitivity studies form an extremely useful guide to therapy and must not be negated by instituting antibiotic therapy prematurely.

192

2. Preoperative Evaluation:

In most instances patients requiring major surgical procedures have additional laboratory studies done in a prophylactic sense to determine the patient's ability to withstand the stress of the procedure. In many institutions, there are well-established screening routines, determined in concert with the consulting anesthesiologist. It is obvious that the selection of these tests rests upon a thorough history and physical examination. It is equally apparent in this regard that the patient who is to have an orthopaedic procedure differs in no way from those patients having other surgical procedures. All patients require an adequate preoperative assessment of their cardiovascular, respiratory, renal, hepatic, endocrine, and hematologic systems to prevent clinically unforeseen but statistically significant complications.

Certain situations are particularly germane to orthopaedic patients and deserve some special mention:

a. Drug History: As many patients who need reconstructive joint procedures have been treated with corticosteroids, they are particularly prone to shock during surgery. Omission of inquiry as to prior steroid therapy and lack of adequate preventative steps unnecessarily jeopardize the patient. A similar situation exists in the elderly hypertensive patient who has been on prolonged anti-hypertensive drug therapy.

b. Bleeding Tendencies: Many diseases of coagulation are manifested by joint pathology and failure to assess bleeding and clotting mechanisms adequately may place the patient in some danger.

c. Respiratory Function: Patients with severe spinal disease, and particularly scoliotic children, may have subclinical respiratory deficits. Due to these deficits and the rather unphysiologic positions during procedures, on the spine, preoperative measurements of vital capacity and blood gases are of considerable help to the patient.

d. Thrombo-embolic Phenomena: Thrombophlebitis and subsequent pulmonary embolization are especially common in postoperative orthopaedic patients because of the frequent necessity for prolonged immobilization combined with the nature of the procedures. In these instances, adequate prophylactic steps should be taken before and after surgery to minimize these serious complications.

There is an infinite number of possibilities of other such problems. That their recognition and investigation cannot be done adequately solely by "routine" preoperative laboratory screening is self-evident.

3. Postoperative and Post-traumatic Monitoring:

The use of the laboratory in monitoring patients following major surgery or severe injury is invaluable. It allows surveillance of blood volume, electrolyte balance, fluid balance, and serial determinations of special studies such as glucose levels in diabetics or prothrombin times in anticoagulated patients.

Judicious monitoring using the laboratory combined with clinical information provides the key to the prevention and treatment of shock, pulmonary edema, dehydration, and pulmonary emboli to name but a few. The key word is "combined" — no routine set of laboratory values by itself will safeguard a patient. Equally important to recognize are the limitations of clinical recognition of acidosis, alkalosis, and similar problems at the time when these problems are reversible or preventable. Without adequate, laboratory data, timely recognition of these conditions is not possible.

APPENDIX

Schema of Ossification of the Skeleton
Total Skeleton

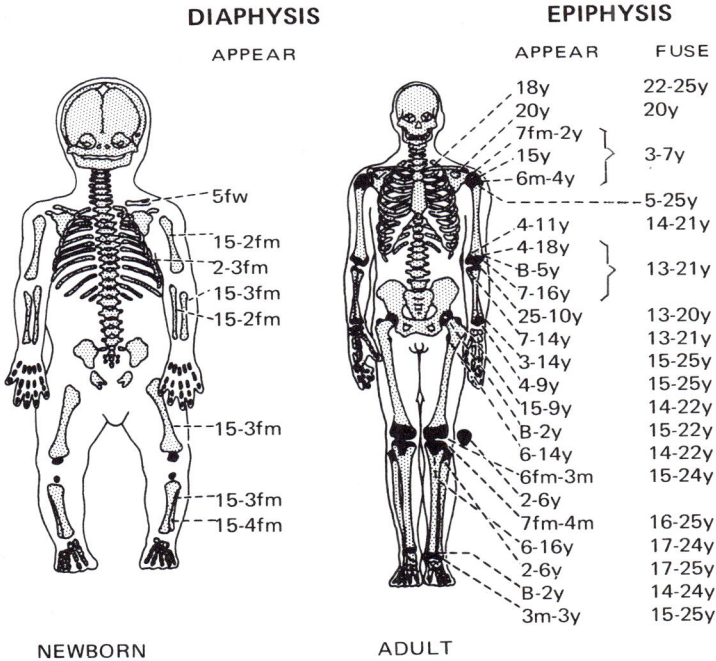

DIAPHYSIS

APPEAR

EPIPHYSIS

	APPEAR	FUSE
	18y	22-25y
	20y	20y
	7fm-2y	
	15y	3-7y
	6m-4y	
		5-25y
	4-11y	14-21y
	4-18y	
	B-5y	13-21y
	7-16y	
	25-10y	13-20y
	7-14y	13-21y
	3-14y	15-25y
	4-9y	15-25y
	15-9y	14-22y
	B-2y	15-22y
	6-14y	14-22y
	6fm-3m	15-24y
	2-6y	
	7fm-4m	16-25y
	6-16y	17-24y
	2-6y	17-25y
	B-2y	14-24y
	3m-3y	15-25y

Diaphysis labels: 5fw, 15-2fm, 2-3fm, 15-3fm, 15-2fm, 15-3fm, 15-3fm, 15-4fm

NEWBORN

ADULT

```
                    LEGEND
    fw—Fetal weeks    fm—Fetal months
       m—Postnatal months    y—Years
```

Fig. 135

195

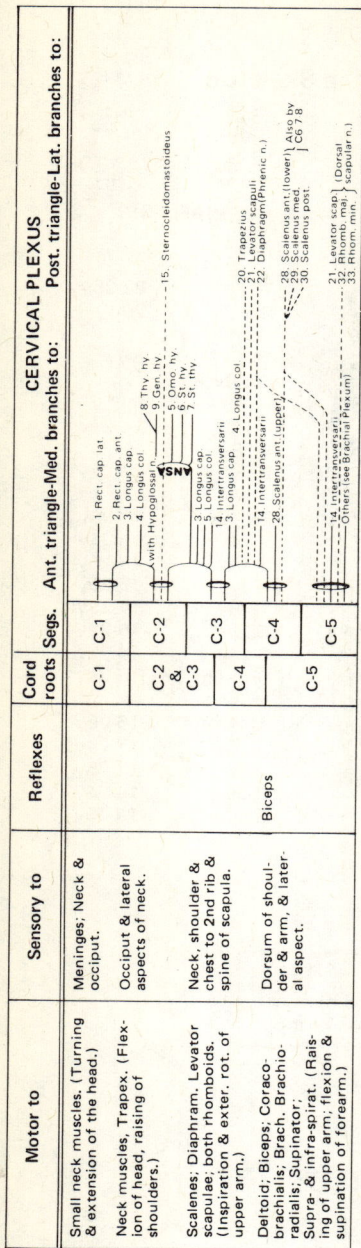

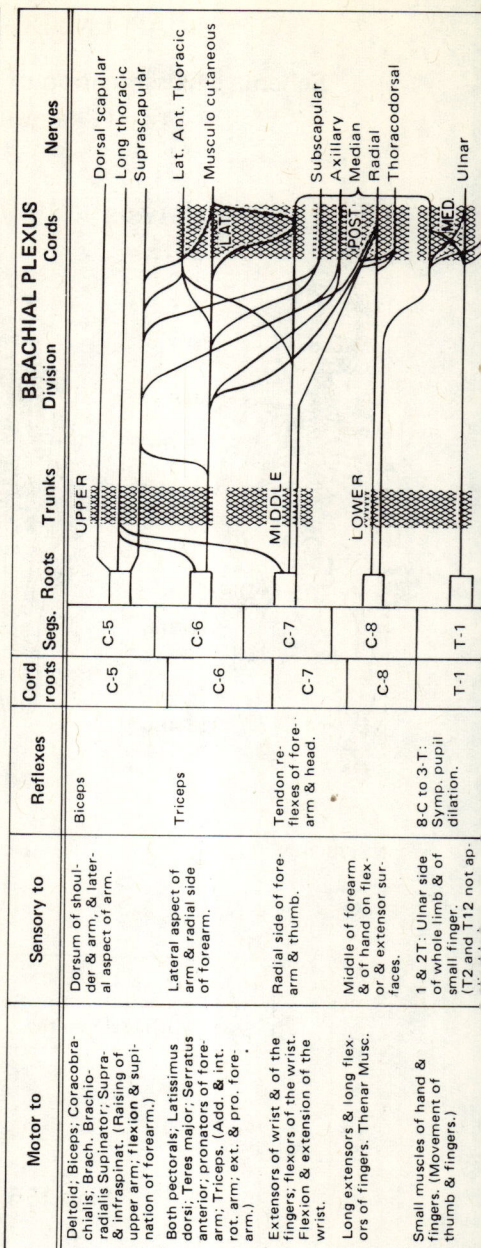

CERVICAL PLEXUS

Motor to	Sensory to	Reflexes	Cord roots	Segs.	Ant. triangle–Med. branches to:	Post. triangle–Lat. branches to:
Small neck muscles. (Turning & extension of the head.)	Meninges; Neck & occiput.		C-1	C-1	1 Rect cap lat	
Neck muscles, Trapex. (Flexion of head, raising of shoulders.)	Occiput & lateral aspects of neck.		C-2 & C-3	C-2	2 Rect cap ant 4 Longus cap with Hypoglossal 8 Thy. hy. 9 Gen. hy. ANSA 5 Omo. hy. 6 St. hy. 7 St. thy.	15. Sternocleidomastoideus
Scalenes; Diaphram, Levator scapulae; both rhomboids. (Inspiration & exter. rot. of upper arm.)	Neck, shoulder & chest to 2nd rib & spine of scapula.			C-3	3 Longus cap. 3 Longus col 4 Intertransversarii 3 Longus cap.	20 Trapezius 21 Levator scapuli 22 Diaphragm(Phrenic n.)
Deltoid; Biceps; Coracobrachialis; Brach. Brachioradialis; Supinator; Supra- & infra-spirat. (Raising of upper arm; flexion & supination of forearm.)	Dorsum of shoulder & arm, & lateral aspect.	Biceps	C-4	C-4	3 Longus col 14 intertransversarii	28 Scalenus ant (upper) 29 Scalenus med. 30 Scalenus post.
			C-5	C-5	14 intertransversarii Others (see Brachial Plexus)	21 Levator scap 32 Rhomb. maj. 33 Rhom. min. {Dorsal scapular n.} Also by C6 7

BRACHIAL PLEXUS

Motor to	Sensory to	Reflexes	Cord roots	Segs.	Roots	Trunks	Division	Cords	Nerves
Deltoid; Biceps; Coracobrachialis; Brach. Brachioradialis Supinator; Supra- & infraspinat. (Raising of upper arm; flexion & supination of forearm.)	Dorsum of shoulder & arm, & lateral aspect of arm.	Biceps	C-5	C-5		UPPER		LAT	Dorsal scapular Long thoracic Suprascapular Lat. Ant. Thoracic Musculo cutaneous
Both pectorals; Latissimus dorsi; Teres major; Serratus anterior; pronators of forearm; Triceps. (Add. & int. rot. arm; ext. & pro. forearm.)	Lateral aspect of arm & radial side of forearm.	Triceps	C-6	C-6		MIDDLE		POST	Subscapular Axillary Median Radial Thoracodorsal
Extensors of wrist & of the fingers; flexors of the wrist. Flexion & extension of the wrist.	Radial side of forearm & thumb.	Tendon reflexes of forearm & head.	C-7	C-7		LOWER		MED	Ulnar
Long extensors & long flexors of fingers. Thenar Musc.	Middle of forearm & of hand on flexor & extensor surfaces.		C-8	C-8					
Small muscles of hand & fingers. (Movement of thumb & fingers.)	1 & 2T: Ulnar side of whole limb & of small finger. (T2 and T12 not ap-	8-C to 3-T: Symp. pupil dilation.	T-1	T-1					

Fig. 136

Motor to	Sensory to	Reflexes	Cord roots	Segs.	LUMBO-SACRAL PLEXUS
Lowermost abdom. muscles; quadratus lumborum; psoas; sartorius.	Outside of gluteal region & inguinal region.	Sympath. urinary bl., 1L.	L1	L1	Ilio-hypogastric / Ilio-inguinal / Genito-femoral; Q.L.
Ilio-psoas; cremaster.	Lat. aspect of thigh; testicles.	Cremaster 1 to 3L.	L2	L2	Ps. maj. & min.; Q.L.
Ilio-psoas; adductors of thigh; quadriceps; int. rot. of thigh. (Flex. int. rot. & adduction of thigh.)	Ant. & inner aspect thigh. Knee.	Patellar, 2 to 4L.	L3	L3	Femoralis; Obturator; Q.L. Ps. min.
Quadriceps. (Extension of leg.)	Inner side of leg & foot; ant. & inside of thigh.	Gluteal, 4 & 5L.	L4	L4	Q.L.
Gluteus med. & min.; semimembr.; semi-tend; biceps; tensor fascia lata; tibialis ant. (Abduct of thigh, flexion of the leg.)	External aspect of leg & foot. External aspect of thigh?		L5	L5	Superior gluteal; Inferior-gluteal; Common peroneal; L-S cord; Ant. / Post.
Gluteus max. (Obturator int. & pyriformis, & gemelli, & quadratus fem. (all extend and rotate the thigh ext.) Tibialis ant. & the peronei, & ext. digit longus (all dorsiflex the foot & toes.)	Post. aspect of thigh; Post. aspect of calf; sole of foot; outer foot border; toes.	Plantar & Achilles, 5L & 2S.	S1	S1	Sciatic; Tibial; Pi. (post.); Ant. / Post.
Gastrocnemius & soleus (large calf m.) Ext. & flex. digit. comm. & hallucis. Tibialis post. Small muscles of foot. (Erection; plantar flex. of foot & toes.)	Saddle area; outside of leg; outer foot border; colon & bladder sensitivity.	Erection.	S2	S2	To adductor magnus (inf.); To Quad. fem. & Gem. inf.; To Obt. int. & Gem. sup.; Inf. hemorr. (to sph. an. ext.); Pi. (post.); Ant.
Perineal m.; striated m. of rectum, ureter, & sex organs; sphincters.	Middle of saddle area; perineum; scrotum; penis.	Ejaculat. Bladder & Rectum, 2 to 5S.	S3	S3	Deep perineal to: L.A. (perin. surf.) / Sph. an. ext. (ant.) / Trans. peri. superf. & prof. / Bulbocavernous / Sph. ureth. memb. / Ischiocavernous; Pudendal nerve
Voluntary initiation of urination & defecation.			S 3-5	S 3-5	To L.A. (pelvic surf.) Coccyg., & Sph. an. ext.
Voluntary initiation or urinat. & defecation.	Perineum, anus, & perianal area.	Anal, 5S.	S 4-5	S 4-5	Perineal nerve to Sph. an. ext (post.)

Abbreviations:
Q.L. = Quadratus lumborum
Ps. = Psoas
Pi. = Piriformis
L.A. = Levator ani

197

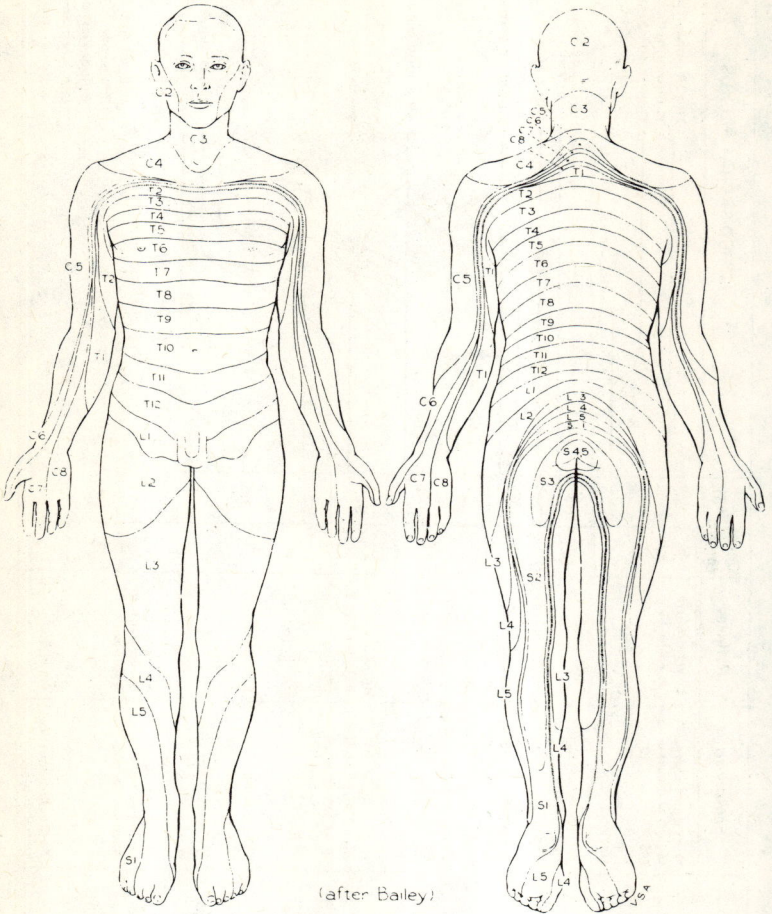

(after Bailey)

Motor - extensor hallicus longus → L5
gastroc-soleus → S1
knee → L4

Fig. 137 Sensory Dermatome Levels

198

AVERAGE RANGES OF JOINT MOTION

	SOURCES				
JOINT	(1)	(2)	(3)	(4)	AVERAGES
ELBOW =					
FLEXION	150	135	150	150	146
HYPEREXTENSION	0	0	0	0	0
FOREARM =					
PRONATION	80	75	50	80	71
SUPINATION	80	85	90	80	84
WRIST =					
EXTENSION	60	65	90	70	71
FLEXION	70	70		80	73
ULNAR DEV.	30	40	30	30	33
RADIAL DEV.	20	20	15	20	19
THUMB =					
ABDUCTION		55	50	70	58
FLEXION					
I-P Jt.	80	75	90	80	81
M — P	60	50	50	50	53
M — C				15	15
EXTENSION					
Distal Jt.		20	10	20	17
M — P		5	10	0	8
M — C				20	20
FINGERS =					
FLEXION					
Distal Jt.	70	70	90	90	80
Middle Jt.	100	100		100	100
Proximal Jt.	90	90		90	90

Fig. 138

199

AVERAGE RANGES OF JOINT MOTION

JOINT	SOURCES				
	(1)	(2)	(3)	(4)	AVERAGES
KNEE =					
FLEXION	120	135	145	135	134
HYPEREXTENSION			10	10	10
ANKLE =					
FLEXION (plantar flexion)	40	50	50	50	48
EXTENSION (dorsiflexion)	20	15	15	20	18
HIND FOOT (subtalar) =					
INVERSION				5	5
EVERSION				5	5
FORE FOOT =					
INVERSION	30	35		35	33
EVERSION	20	20		15	18
TOES =					
GREAT TOE					
I-P Jt.					
Flexion	30			90	60
Extension	0			0	0
Proximal Jt.					
Flexion	30	35		45	37
Extension	50	70		70	63
2nd TO 5th TOES =					
FLEXION					
Distal Jt.	50			60	55
Middle Jt.	40			35	38
Proximal Jt.	30			40	35
Extension	40			40	40

Fig. 139

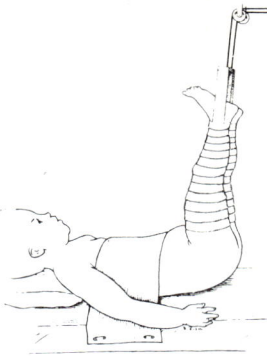

Bryant's Traction

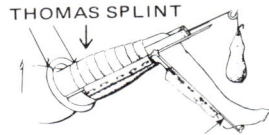

THOMAS SPLINT

Pearson Attachment

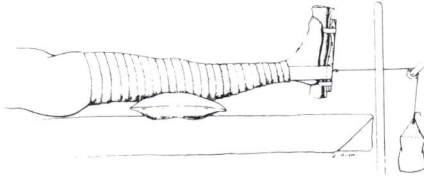

Buck's Extension

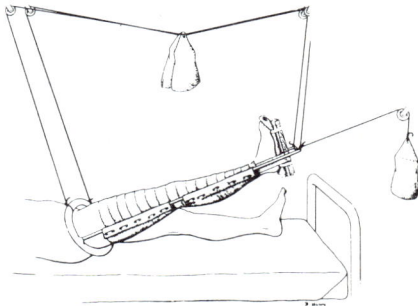

Suspended or Floating Traction

Fig. 140

201

INDEX OF ORTHOPAEDIC TERMINOLOGY

Order Blank

Enclosed please find Check   for $ _____
                      M.O.

Please ship _____ copies of "Manual of Orthopaedic Surgery" at $5.00 per copy, including shipping
charges.*

Name _____

Address _____

City, State, Zip _____

Make checks payable in U.S. Funds
and Mail Orders to:

**American Orthopaedic Association
444 North Michigan Avenue
Chicago, Illinois 60611**

*15% discount on order for ten (10) or more copies.